The Mediterranean Dash Diet Cookbook

2 Books In 1

How To Improve Your Health And Lose Weight With Easy, Healthy Delicious Recipes For Living And Eating Well Every Day!

Marla Smith

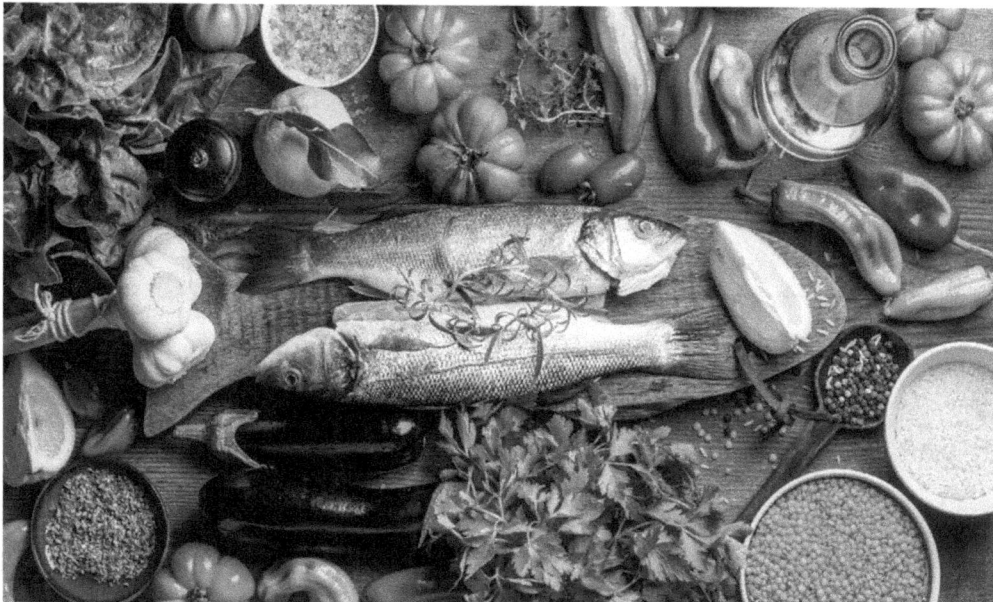

Table of Contents

Mediterranean Diet For Beginners 2020

Introduction 13

Chapter 1 What is the Mediterranean diet? 14

The Mediterranean Diet Pyramid 14

Chapter 2 The History of the Mediterranean diet 22

Chapter 3 The Science Behind the Mediterranean Diet 25

Chapter 4 The Mediterranean Lifestyle 28

Chapter 5 Health Benefits of the Mediterranean Diet 30

How the Mediterranean diet works 30

Chapter 6 Step by Step Instructions to Roll Out the Improvement 35

Chapter 7 A Delicious Path to Weight Loss 37

Chapter 8 Essential Mediterranean Food 42

Fruits & Vegetables 42

Whole Grains 42

Using Olive Oil 42

Fish & Chicken 43

Nuts 43

Red Wine 43

Spices 43

Dairy 44

Legumes 44

Foods to Avoid 44

Swapping Food Out..45

The Take Away 45

Chapter 9 Planning Your Mediterranean Diet..............................**46**

A proportionate combination of elements 46

Understand the importance of whole products.......................46

Elements to be considered by Mediterranean Diet enthusiasts 46

Chapter 10 21-Day Meal Plan **49**

Chapter 11 Breakfast & Brunch Recipes............................**53**

Breakfast Egg on Avocado...53

Breakfast Egg-artichoke Casserole 53

Brekky Egg-potato Hash 55

Dill and Tomato Frittata 56

Paleo Almond Banana Pancakes 57

Banana-Coconut Breakfast..58

Basil and Tomato Soup 59

Butternut Squash Hummus 60

Cajun Jambalaya Soup 61

Collard Green Wrap Greek Style 62

Portobello Mushroom Pizza 64

Roasted Root Veggies 64

Amazingly Good Parsley Tabbouleh 65

Appetizing Mushroom Lasagna 66

Artichokes, Olives & Tuna Pasta 68

Baked Ricotta With Pears...70

Mediterranean Fruit Bulgur Breakfast Bowl 71

Scrambled Eggs With Goat Cheese And Roasted Peppers 72

Marinara Eggs With Parsley..73

Italian Breakfast Bruschetta 74

Julene's Green Juice..75

Chapter 12 Lunch Recipes..76

Italian Lamb Shanks 76

Beef Goulash 78

Instant Pot Korean Beef 79

Beef Ragu 80

Sloppy Joe with Beef...81

Beef & Tomato Soup...83

Ground Lamb Curry 84

Rosemary Lamb 86

Thyme Lamb 87

Garlic Lamb Shanks with Port 88

Sea Bass in a Pan with Peppers 89

Crusty Tuna Patties 91

Baked Teriyaki Salmon 92

Whole Roasted Mackerel 94

White Fish sautéed with Lemon, Capers and Herbs 95

Baked Fish with Olives, Tomatoes, and Eggplant 96

Grilled White Fish with Fresh Basil Pesto 97

White Fish with Chickpeas and Chorizo 98

Fresh Salmon with Lemon Butter and New Potatoes...99

Fresh Fish Puttanesca Salad with Couscous...100

Tuna Croquettes 101

Chapter 13 Dinner Recipes..**104**

Stuffed Sardines 104

Mini Greek Meatloaves 105

Yogurt-And-Herb-Marinated Pork Tenderloin 106

Rosemary Potatoes 108

Delicious Italian Bell Pepper...108

Pesto Zucchini..109

Pesto Cauliflower..110

Italian Tomato Mushrooms 112

Chickpea & Potato...113

Zesty Green Beans...114

Walnut-Rosemary Crusted Salmon 115

Caprese Stuffed Portobello Mushrooms......................................116

Greek Salad Nachos 117

Greek Chicken with Lemon Vinaigrette and Roasted Spring Vegetables118

Chicken in Tomato-Balsamic Pan Sauce 119

Chicken Souvlaki Kebabs with Mediterranean Couscous 121

Caprese Chicken Hasselback style 122

Simple Grilled Salmon with Veggies..123

Greek Turkey Burgers with Spinach, Feta &Tzatziki.....................124

Mediterranean Chicken Quinoa Bowl 125

Creamy Dill Potatoes...127

Chapter 14 Snacks Recipes..**129**

Mediterranean Flatbread with Toppings 129

Smoked Salmon and Goat Cheese Bites 130

Mediterranean Chickpea Bowl...131

Hummus Snack Bowl...133

Crock-Pot Paleo Chunky Mix..134

Smoked Eggplant Dip 135

Savory Spinach Feta and Sweet Pepper Muffins 137

Italian Oven Roasted Vegetables 138

Greek Spinach Yogurt Artichoke Dip 139

Sautéed Apricots...140

Spiced Kale Chips 141

Yogurt Dip... 142

Zucchini Fritters 143

Easy Hummus.. 144

Cucumber Bites 144

Stuffed Avocado 145

Wrapped Plums 146

Cucumber Sandwich Bites 146

Cucumber Rolls 147

Olives and Cheese Stuffed Tomatoes.. 148

Tomato Salsa 148

Chapter 15 Dessert Recipes...150

Blueberries Stew.. 150

Mandarin Cream 150

Creamy Mint Strawberry Mix 151

Vanilla Cake 152

Pumpkin Cream 153

Chia and Berries Smoothie Bowl 153

Minty Coconut Cream 154

Watermelon Cream.. 155

Grapes Stew... 155

Cocoa Sweet Cherry Cream 156

Loukoumade (Fried Honey Balls).. 156

Crème Caramel 158

Galaktoboureko 159

Kourabiedes Almond Cookies... 160

Ekmek Kataifi 161

Revani Syrup Cake 163

Almonds and Oats Pudding 164

Chocolate Cups...165

Mango Bowls 165

Cocoa and Pears Cream...166

Pineapple Pudding 167

Conclusion **168**

Dash Diet Cookbook

Introduction **170**

What is the DASH Diet? **171**

Why The Dash Diet Works 171

DASH Diet Health Plan 172

Dash diet for weight loss 173

Steps towards Transitioning to the DASH Diet 174

Benefits of the DASH Diet **175**

Cardiovascular Health 175

Helpful for Patients with Diabetes 175

Weight Reduction...176

Importance of Healthy Weight...**178**

Health Benefits of Consuming Good Fats **181**

Dash Food Groups Intake...183

Enhance your Results with Exercise....................................**186**

Breakfast Recipes **192**

Sweet Avocado Smoothie 192

Cinnamon Apple Overnight Oats 192

Blueberry Muffins 193

Yogurt & Banana Muffins...194

Berry Quinoa Bowls 195

Pineapple Green Smoothie 196

Peanut Butter & Banana Smoothie 197

Mushroom Frittata 197

Cheesy Omelet 198

Ginger Congee 199

Egg Melts 200

Fluffy Pancakes for Breakfast 201

Fluffy Zucchini Bread 202

Spinach Crustless Quiche 203

Friendly French Toast 204

Everyday Crepes 205

Hash Brown Cheesy Ham Casserole 206

Baffle Waffles 207

Banana Sour Cream Bread 208

Cinnamon Baked Bread 209

Buttermilk Pancake 211

French Toast with Blueberries 212

Plumpy Pumpkin Bread 214

Vintage Pancakes 215

Pampered Zucchini Bread 216

Lunch Recipes 219

Shrimp Quesadillas 219

The OG Tuna Sandwich 219

Easy To Understand Mussels 220

Chili-Rubbed Tilapia with Asparagus & Lemon 221

Parmesan-Crusted Fish 222

Lemony Braised Beef Roast 223

Grilled Fennel-cumin Lamb Chops 224

Beef Heart...224

Jerk Beef and Plantain Kabobs 225

Beef Pot 226

Cheesy Black Bean Wraps 227

Arugula Risotto 228

Vegetarian Stuffed Eggplant 229

Vegetable Tacos 230

Fruit Chicken Salad 231

Whole Grain Pasta with Meat Sauce 233

Beef Tacos 234

Dirty Rice 235

Beef with Pea Pods..237

Whole-Grain Rotini with Ground Pork 237

Roasted Pork Loin with Herbs 238

Garlic Lime Pork Chops...239

Lamb Curry with Tomatoes and Spinach......................240

Pomegranate-Marinated Leg of Lamb 241

Beef Fajitas with Peppers 243

Dinner Recipes..**245**

Pork Medallions with Herbs de Provence 245

Baked Chicken 245

Orange Chicken and Broccoli Stir-Fry..........................246

Mediterranean Lemon Chicken and Potatoes...............247

Tandoori Chicken 248

Mighty Garlic and Butter Sword Fish 249

Supreme Cooked Lobster 250

Tilapia with Parsley...250

Thai Coconut Tilapia and Rice..251

Nutmeg Pork Chops 252

Butter and Dill Pork Chops 253

Paprika Pork with Carrots 254

Pork and Greens Mix..255

Sage Pork Chops 256

Pork with Avocados 256

Simple Roast..257

Easy Chili 258

Italian Shrimp Dinner 259

Cabbage & Beef Stew 260

Fish Curry 261

Beef Bourguignon 262

Lobster Bisque..263

Pineapple Spicy Shrimp 264

Seafood & Chickpea Pot 265

Chicken & Mushroom Stew 266

Side Dish Recipes..268

Apple & Barley Side 268

Spinach Dip 268

Rice & Endives..269

Lentils & Peas 270

Leeks & Fennel 271

Summer Squash Ribbons with Lemon and Ricotta..271

Sautéed Kale with Tomato and Garlic 272

Roasted Broccoli with Tahini Yogurt Sauce..273

Green Beans with Pine Nuts and Garlic 274

Roasted Harissa Carrots 275

Cucumbers with Feta, Mint, and Sumac 276

Cherry Tomato Bruschetta 277

Roasted Red Pepper Hummus...278

Baked Eggplant Baba Ganoush 279

White Bean Romesco Dip 281

Roasted Cherry Tomato Caprese..282

Italian Crepe with Herbs and Onion..284

Pita Pizza with Olives, Feta, and Red Onion 285

Roasted Za'atar Chickpeas 287

Roasted Rosemary Olives 288

Crispy Cinnamon Apple Chips..289

Coconut Date Energy Bites 290

Roasted Root Vegetable Chips with French Onion Yogurt Dip 290

Stovetop Cheese Popcorn 292

Sweet & Salty Nut Mix 293

Dessert Recipes 296

Easy Cinnamon Baked Apples..296

Chocolate Cake In a Mug 296

Peanut Butter Banana "Ice Cream" 297

Banana-Cashew Cream Mousse 298

Peach and Blueberry Tart 299

Sriracha Parsnip Fries..300

Tortilla Strawberry Chips 301

Almond Rice Pudding 302

Sweet Potatoes and Apples Mix...303

Sautéed Bananas with Orange Sauce 304

Caramelized Blood Oranges with Ginger Cream...............................305

Grilled Minted Watermelon 306

Caramelized Apricot Pots..307

Melon Mojito Granita..308

Mocha Pops 309

Rhubarb Pie 310

Berry No Bake Bars 311

Tropical Fruit Napoleon 312

Ginger Peach Pie 313

Mocha Ricotta Cream..315

Fresh Parfait 316

Toasted Almond Ambrosia 317

Apple Dumplings 317

Apricot Biscotti 319

Apple & Berry Cobbler 321

Conclusion...**323**

Mediterranean Diet For Beginners 2020

All You Need to Know About the Mediterranean Diet to Start Losing Weight and Improve your Health. Reset your Body Through Simple and Delicious Recipes!

Marla Smith

Introduction

In this book, you'll learn everything you need to get started on the Mediterranean diet. The Mediterranean diet is all about living well and eating like the people of the Mediterranean. This includes vegetables, grains, legumes, dairy, eggs, poultry and smaller amounts of red meat. It's about dining with friends, moderate physical activity, and food that will lift your spirits. It's all about eating the traditional food of the countries that make up the Mediterranean, including Italy, Spain, France, Greece, Israel, and even Turkey. This diet promotes overall health, including weight loss, and it's great at helping reduce the risk of Parkinson's, Alzheimer's, promoting heart health, and reducing the risk of cancer.

With the Mediterranean Diet you'll have foods that are based on vegetable, fruits, grains, olive oil, nuts, beans, legumes, herbs, spices and seeds. You'll consume fish and seafood often, with cheese, yogurt and other dairy products in moderation. Poultry and eggs are allowed in moderation, but you shouldn't eat them more than twice a week. Other meats and sweets should be eaten rarely, and drinking water is encouraged. Say goodbye to sodas, and replace it with a glass of red wine in the evenings and water to hydrate. While physical activity isn't required on this diet, at least moderate activity is encouraged if you to get the most out of the Mediterranean lifestyle. Even taking an evening stroll can help to elevate the effects of the diet, including weight loss.

Chapter 1

What is the Mediterranean diet?

The Mediterranean diet refers to the traditional eating habits and lifestyles of people living around the Mediterranean Sea – Italy, Spain, France, Greece, and some North African countries. The Mediterranean diet has become very popular in recent times, as people from these regions have better health and suffer from fewer ailments, such as cancer and cardiovascular issues. Food plays a key role in this.

Research has uncovered the many benefits of this diet. According to the results of a 2013 study, many overweight and diabetic patients showed a surprising improvement in their cardiovascular health after eating the Mediterranean diet for 5 years. The study was conducted among 7000 people in Spain. There was a marked 30% reduction in cardiovascular disease in this high-risk group.

The report took the world by storm after the New England Journal of Medicine published the findings. Several studies have indicated its many health benefits – the Mediterranean diet may stabilize the level of blood sugar, prevent Alzheimer's disease, reduce the risk of heart disease and stroke, improve brain health, ease anxiety and depression, promote weight loss, and even lower the risk of certain types of cancer.

The diet differs from country to country, and even within the regions of these countries because of cultural, ethnic, agricultural, religious, and economic differences. So there is no one standard Mediterranean diet. However, there are several common factors.

The Mediterranean Diet Pyramid

The Med diet food pyramid is a nutrition guide to help people eat the right foods in the correct quantities and the prescribed frequency as per the traditional eating habits of people from the Mediterranean coast countries.

The pyramid was developed by the World Health Organization, Harvard School of Public Health, and the old ways Preservation Trust in 1993.

There are 6 food layers in the pyramid with physical activity at the base, which is an important element to maintain a healthy life.

Just above it is the first food layer, consisting of whole grains, breads, beans, pasta, and nuts. It is the strongest layer having foods that are recommended by the Mediterranean diet. Next comes fruits and vegetables. As you move up the pyramid, you will find foods that must be eaten less and less, with the topmost layer consisting of foods that should be avoided or restricted.

The Mediterranean diet food pyramid is easy to understand. It provides an easy way to follow the eating plan.

The Food Layers

1. **Whole Grains, Breads, Beans** – *The lowest and the widest layer with foods that are strongly recommended. Your meals should be made of mostly these items. Eat whole-wheat bread, whole-wheat pita, whole-grain roll and bun, whole-grain cereal, whole-wheat pasta, and brown rice. 4 t0 6 servings a day will give you plenty of nutrition.*

2. **Fruits, Vegetables** – *Almost as important as the lowest layer. Eat non-starchy vegetables daily like asparagus, broccoli, beets, tomatoes, carrots, cucumber, cabbage, cauliflower, turnips 4 to 8 servings daily. Take 2 to 4 servings of fruits every day. Choose seasonal fresh fruits.*

3. **Olive oil** – *Cook your meals preferably in extra-virgin olive oil. Daily consumption. Healthy for the body, it lowers the low-density lipoprotein cholesterol (LDL) and total cholesterol level. Up to 2 tablespoons of olive oil is allowed. The diet also allows canola oil.*

4. **Fish** – *Now we come to the food layers that have to be consumed weekly and not daily. You can have fish 2 to 3 times a week. Best is fatty sea fish like tuna, herring, salmon, and sardines. Sea fish will give you heart-healthy omega-3 fatty acids and plenty of proteins. Shellfish, including mussels, oysters, shrimp, and clams are also good.*

5. **Poultry, cheese, yogurt** – *The diet should include cheese, yogurt, eggs, chicken, and other poultry products, but in moderation. Maximum 2-3 times in a week. Low-fat dairy is best. Soy milk, cheese, or yogurt is better.*

. Meats, sweets – *This is the topmost layer consisting of foods that are best avoided. You can have them once or twice in a month max. Remember, the Mediterranean diet is plant-based. There is very little room for meat, especially red meat. If you cannot live without it, then take red meat in small portions. Choose lean cuts. Have sweets only to celebrate. For instance, you can have a couple of sweets after following the diet for a month.*

Recommended Foods

For example, most people living in the region eat a diet rich in whole grains, vegetables, fruits, nuts, seeds, fish, fats, and legumes. It is not a restrictive diet like the many low-fat eating plans. Actually, fat is encouraged, but only from healthy sources, such as polyunsaturated fat (omega-3 fatty acids) that you will get from fish and monounsaturated fat from olive oil.

It is strongly plant-based, but not exclusively vegetarian. The diet recommends limiting the intake of saturated fats and trans fats that you get from red meat and processed foods. You must also limit the intake of dairy products.

• Fruits and vegetables – Eat daily. Try to have 7-10 servings every day. Meals are strongly based on plant-based foods. Eat fresh fruits and vegetables. Pick from seasonal varieties.

• Whole grains – Eat whole-grain cereal, bread, and pasta. All parts of whole grains – the germ, bran, and the endosperm provide healthy nutrients. These nutrients are lost when the grain is refined into white flour.

• Healthy fats only – Avoid butter for cooking. Switch to olive oil. Dip your bread in flavored olive oil instead of applying margarine or butter on bread. Trans fats and saturated fats can cause heart disease.

• Fish – Fish is encouraged. Eat fatty fish like herring, mackerel, albacore tuna, sardines, lake trout, and salmon. Fatty fish will give you plenty of healthy omega-3 fatty acids that reduce inflammations. Omega-3 fatty acids also reduced blood clotting, decreased triglycerides, and improves heart health. Eat fresh seafood two times a week. Avoid deep-fried fish. Choose grilled fish.

- Legumes – Provides the body with minerals, protein, complex carbohydrates, polyunsaturated fatty acids, and fiber. Eat daily.

- Dairy and poultry – You can eat eggs, milk products, and chicken throughout the week, but with moderation. Restrict cheese. Go for plain or low-fat Greek yogurt instead of cheese.

- Nuts and seeds – 3 or more servings every week. Eat a variety of nuts, seeds, and beans. Walnuts and almonds are all allowed.

- Red meat – The Mediterranean diet is not meat-based. You can still have red meat, but only once or twice a week max. If you love red meat, then make sure that it is lean. Take small portions only. Avoid processed meats like salami, sausage, and bologna.

- Olive Oil – The key source of fat. Olive oil will give you monounsaturated fat that lowers the LDL or low-density lipoprotein cholesterol and total cholesterol level. Seeds and nuts will also provide you monounsaturated fat. You can also have canola oil but no cream, butter, mayonnaise, or margarine. Take up to 4 tablespoons of olive oil a day. For best results, only take extra-virgin olive oil.

- Wine – Red wine is allowed, but with moderation. Don't take more than a glass of red wine daily. Best take only 3-4 days a week.

- Desserts – Say no to ice cream, sweets, pies, and chocolate cake. Fresh fruits are good.

Main Components –

- Focus on natural foods – Avoid processed foods as much as you can

- Be flexible – Plan to have a variety of foods

- Consume fruits, vegetables, healthy fats, and whole grains daily

- Have weekly plans for poultry, fish, eggs, and beans

- Take dairy products moderately

- Limit red meat intake

- Take water instead of soda. Only take wine when you are having a meal.

Foods in the Traditional Mediterranean Diet

Whole Grains	Vegetables	Fruits	Protein	Dairy	Others
Brown rice	Artichokes	Apples	Almonds	Low/non-fat plain or Greek yogurt	Bay leaf
Oats	Arugula	Apricots	Walnuts	Manchego cheese	Basil
Bulgur	Beats	Avocados	Pistachios	Brie cheese	Olive oil
Barley	Broccoli	Figs	Cannellini Beans	Ricotta cheese	Red wine
Farrow	Cucumbers	Olives	Chickpeas	Parmesan cheese	Mint
Wheat berries	Eggplant	Strawberries	Kidney beans	Feta cheese	Pepper
Pasta	Onions	Tomatoes	Salmon		cumin

Whole grain bread	Spinach	Melons	Tuna		Garlic
Couscous	Potatoes	Grapes	Eggs		Anise spice

Foods Allowed

You should consume plenty of fruits, vegetables, nuts, seeds, beans, whole grains, herbs, and legumes. Olive oil and canola oil are both allowed.

Eat Moderately

Fish, seafood, chicken, eggs, low-fat cheese, and yogurt.

Restricted Foods

This list includes refined grains like white rice, white bread, sweets, baked products, and soda. Also, restrict processed meats and red meat. Watch out for high-fat dairy products like butter and ice cream and trans-fats in margarine and processed foods.

Med Diet Serving Sizes

Food Groups and Daily/Weekly Servings	Serving Sizes
Non-starchy vegetables – 4 to 8 servings	1 serving is ½ cup of cooked vegetables or 1 cup of raw vegetables Asparagus, artichoke, broccoli, beets, Brussels sprouts, cabbage, celery, cauliflower, carrots, eggplant, tomatoes, cucumber, onion, zucchini, turnips, mushrooms, and salad greens and. Note: Peas, corn, and potatoes are starchy vegetables.

Fruits – 2 to 4 servings	One serving is a small fruit or ½ cup juice or ¼ cup dried fruit Eat fresh fruits for their nutrients and fiber. You can also have canned fruits with their juice and frozen fruits without added sugar.
Legumes, Nuts, Seeds – 2 to 4 servings	Legumes – 1 serving is ½ cup cooked kidney, pinto, garbanzo, soy, navy beans, lentils, or split peas, or ¼ cup fat-free beans. Nuts and Seeds – 1 serving is 2 tablespoons of sesame or sunflower seeds, 1 tablespoon peanut butter, 7-8 pecans or walnuts, 12-15 almonds, 20 peanuts. Take 1-2 servings of nuts or seeds and 1-2 servings of legumes. Legumes will give you minerals, fiber, and protein, whole nuts provide unsaturated fat without increasing your LDL cholesterol levels.
Low-Fat Dairy – 2 to 3 servings	1 serving is 1 cup of skim milk, non-fat yogurt, or 1 oz. low-fat cheese Replace dairy products with soy yogurt, calcium-rich soy milk, or soy cheese. You need a vitamin D and calcium supplement if you are taking less than 2 servings daily.
Fish – 2 to 3 times a week	One serving is 3 ounces Bake, sauté, roast, broil, poach, or grill. It is best to eat fatty fish, such as sardines, herring, salmon, or mackerel. Fish will provide you omega-3 fats, which offers many health benefits.
Poultry – 1 to 3 times a week	One serving is 3 ounces Sauté, bake, grill, or stir fry the poultry. Eat without the skin.

Whole grains, starchy vegetables – 4 to 6 servings	One serving is 1 ounce of – ½ cup sweet potatoes, potatoes, corn, or peas 1 slice of whole-wheat bread 1 small whole-grain roll ½ large whole-grain bun 6 whole-grain crackers 6-inch whole wheat pita ½ cup cooked brown rice, whole-wheat pasta, or barley ½ cup whole-grain cereal (cracked wheat, oatmeal, quinoa) Whole grains provide fiber and keep the stomach full, promoting weight loss.
Healthy fats – 4 to 6 servings	One serving is – 1 tablespoon of regular salad dressing 2 tablespoons of light salad dressing 2 teaspoons light margarine 1 teaspoon canola or olive oil 1 teaspoon regular mayonnaise 1/8 avocado 5 olives These are mostly unsaturated fats, so your LDL cholesterol levels won't increase.
Alcohol	Men – Max 2 drinks a day. Women – Max 1 drink a day. 1 drink = 4 ounces of wine, 12-ounce beer, or 1-1/2-ounces liquor (vodka, whiskey, brandy, etc.). Avoid alcohol if you have high triglycerides or high BP.

Chapter 2

The History of the Mediterranean diet

Just like it sounds, the Mediterranean diet comes from the dietary traditions of the people of the Mediterranean isle region such as the Romans and Greeks. The people of these regions had a rich diet full of fruits, bread, wine, olive oil, nuts, and seafood. Despite the fatty elements in their diet, the people of this region tended to live longer and overall healthy lives with relatively less cardiovascular heart issues. This phenomenon was noticed by American scientist Ancel Keys in the 1950s.

Keys was an academic researcher at the University of Minnesota in the 1950s who researched healthy eating habits and how to reverse the decline in American cardiovascular health. He found in his research that poor people in the Mediterranean region of the world were healthier compared to the rich American population which had seen a recent rise in cardiovascular heart issues and obesity. Compared to wealthy New Yorkers, the lower class in the Mediterranean lived well into their 90s and tended to be physically active in their senior years. Keys and his team of scientists decided to travel the world and study the link between the region's diet and the health of the people who lived there. In 1957, he traveled and studied the lifestyles, nutrition, exercise, and diet of the United States, Italy, Holland, Greece, Japan, Finland, and Yugoslavia. Twenty years later, he published his findings in a landmark study called "The Seven Countries Study." It evaluated the diets and lifestyles of these regions.

Keys' research found that the dietary choices of the people from the Mediterranean region allowed them to live a longer lifespan and one that kept them more physically active compared to other world populations. The people of Greece, in particular, ate a diet that consisted of healthy fats like seafood, nuts, olive oil, and fatty fish. Despite the amount of fat in these sources, their cardiovascular health stayed consistent without the risk factors for a heart attack or stroke. His study became a guideline for the United States to set its own nutritional standards, and he became known as the father of nutritional science.

With Keys' work leading the way, further research and clinical trials have been conducted on the Mediterranean diet which gives evidence for its health-improving properties. Not only will you lose weight, but you could lower your LDL "bad" cholesterol, lower your blood pressure, and decrease and stabilize blood sugar levels. With a decrease in these signs of cardiovascular heart disease, you can greatly reduce your risk of suffering from heart attack, stroke, or premature death.

It's important to point out that the Mediterranean diet cannot alone bring about these changes to someone's health. It will depend on a variety of other factors in their lifestyle such as genetics, physical exercise, smoking, obesity, drug use, etc. Part of the combination of the Mediterranean diet is incorporating physical exercise into your life. That's how it goes from the Mediterranean "diet" to a Mediterranean "lifestyle" that truly mimics the people of that region. The people of Greece tend to live an active lifestyle with some sort of daily physical activity they partake in. Whether that is walking, sailing, rowing, swimming, or hiking, coupling that physical exercise that with a healthy plant-based diet is what can bring about the beneficial health results. In our current environment, physical activity could mean a session at the gym or even just a walk around the block. It doesn't have to highly intensive, but the important part is incorporating some sort of physical activity in your day, so you can truly gain the benefits of following this diet.

Before we begin listing a rudimentary list of what you can and cannot eat, it's important to highlight that the Mediterranean region consists of many countries with their own unique dietary choices. With this diversity comes many varieties of recipes that you can incorporate into your dishes as long as you are still following the healthy tenets of the Mediterranean diet. This gives a basic outline of which foods you should include on your shopping list and then you can look for recipes from there! What does the basic Mediterranean diet look like?

- Your diet should consist heavily of whole grain bread, extra virgin olive oil, fresh fruits and vegetables, herbs and spices, nuts and seeds, fish and seafood
- You should moderately eat: poultry, cheese, egg, yogurt
- You should try to rarely eat: red meat and organ meat

- You should avoid the following: processed snacks, refined oils (canola oil or vegetable oil), refined grains (white bread), sugary drinks (juice, soda), processed meats (hot dogs, sausages, bacon), trans fats
- You should drink: water, wine

Chapter 3

The Science Behind the Mediterranean Diet

Most of the benefits of this form of diet come from a large number of plant foods associated with the diet. By incorporating a large number of fresh fruits and fresh vegetables in your diet, you are getting a high number of antioxidants and free radicals which are helpful for your body's cellular system and metabolism. The high intake of vitamins, minerals, and fiber you're getting from these plant sources can lower your risk of diabetes, constipation and bowel issues, and heart disease.

Since we've mentioned the Mediterranean diet's intake of healthy fats, it's important to go over why these are healthier for the body. Most of the fat is monounsaturated such as the fat you get from olive oil. This fat, found in nuts, seeds, and oil, tends to be healthier for the body compared to the saturated fat that is found in meat and poultry. A high amount of saturated fat is what tends to wreak havoc on the body's cholesterol and blood pressure.

By staying low in red meat intake, the Mediterranean diet harnesses protein sources from fish and seafood which are healthier for the body. They are high in omega 3 fatty acids. The research regarding omega 3 fatty acids is recent, covering the last 20 to 30 years, but it's shown to be an essential element for vision and brain health, as well as fetal health if a woman is pregnant. Adults are advised to consume at least 250 to 500 milligrams of fatty acids a day. Since most of us don't eat fish every day, you can get in the form of a fish oil supplement. With the Mediterranean diet, that won't be as necessary. The people of the Mediterranean had easy access to fishing and considered fresh fish and seafood a staple in their diet. Not only are there so many varieties, but it also is much healthier for you than having red meat many times a week which tends to raise your cholesterol and clog your arteries. You can still have red meat on this diet, but you should try to consume it more rarely and be aware of your portion sizes. And if you do have red meat, you want to ensure that you are also having healthy vegetables or whole grains along with it.

Along with food, it's important to note that drinking alcohol in moderation is a big part of the Mediterranean diet. Recent studies in the last decade have shown that moderate consumption of red wine could considerably lessen the risk of heart related diseases, gallstones, and diabetes (Type 2). It's believed that red wine contains a component called resveratrol which has health benefits in animals and humans. With this consumption, it's important to note that it is to be moderate, about a glass a day for women, and 2 for men. But with it can come health dangers for pregnant women or birth defects in babies. Many declare alcohol consumption as optional in the diet because some people may be restricted due to health or religious reasons.

We can't speak about the science behind the Mediterranean diet without speaking in length about extra virgin olive oil. With the abundance of olives in the Mediterranean region, olive oil is essential for all their cooking needs. That includes baking, seasoning, frying, and as a fat element in salad vinaigrettes. But when it comes to olive oil, the best oil will be labeled as "extra virgin" because it is the most unprocessed version of olive oil, so the purest that is available. There are many components in extra virgin olive oil that make it such a healthy substance. It contains a high amount of vitamin E which has anti-inflammatory properties for the body. It also has a high amount of phenol substances which contains similar health properties. Oleic acid is another property that is healthy for the heart. It's present in significant amounts in olive oil as compared to other oil types. When it comes to the properties of olive oil, it's taken very seriously by the culinary community. There's an International Olive Council that tests the levels of phenol and acidity in different brands of olive oil to ensure they qualify for the label of "extra virgin". The rule when it comes to olive oil is to go with the old saying "quality over quantity." Most nutritionists will say that consuming 4 to 5 tbsp of olive oil a day should be enough for all your cooking needs. That includes salad dressings, pan frying, baking, or seasoning your food. Olive oil should be kept away from direct sunlight and heat to avoid degradation of the oil.

When we see all these qualities of the Mediterranean diet and how they play out for the body, it's easy to see how this diet can help you improve your health. By including exercise in your routine, you are also gaining the possibility of better health and strengthening your heart and losing more weight. Along with the health benefits possible, the ease of the Mediterranean diet appeals to many people. No counting calories, no measuring food portions, or keeping track of your daily macronutrients. With this flexibility and simply knowing the right foods to eat and avoid, the Mediterranean can be a very easy lifestyle to follow if you are hoping to improve your health.

Chapter 4

The Mediterranean Lifestyle

Not just the food, but the correct lifestyle is also equally important. This includes both getting adequate exercise and making social connections.

Physical Activity – It is at the base of the food pyramid, even lower than the first and most important food layer – getting adequate physical activity is essential. This includes exercising regularly, swimming, biking, running, and playing an active sport. However, there are other ways as well to maintain good health.

You will find many from the Mediterranean region not going to the gym. But, they are not inactive. Many are into a lot of manual labor. They will walk to their workplace, to the bakery, or the farmer's market. They walk to their friend's home. Even a daily walk and moderate exercise will help. Natural movements are good. Avoid the escalator. Take the stairs instead.

How much exercising is good? Working out is always good for health. You don't have to lift weights, though. 10-15 minutes on the treadmill and gym bike 5 days a week should be good. Half an hour of moderate-intensity activity will do. Nothing better if you can also do a few muscle-strengthening activities twice a week. You can also try walking 200 minutes a week or even gardening for an hour 4-5 times a week.

Cook at Home – Home cooked food is always healthier than eating out. For example, restaurant cooked pasta will have higher portions of sodium. Again, you can have one portion of whole-grain spaghetti with tomato sauce and spinach instead of the heavy cream sauce. You can control the ingredients by preparing the meals at home. Home cooked meals have lots of minerals, vitamins, and fiber, and are lower in added sugar, sodium, and saturated fat.

Eat Together – The mealtime should be a social experience. Eating together with friends or family is a great stress buster. It will boost your mood, which will have a positive impact on your physical health. Plus, it will prevent you from overeating too. You will often find the Mediterranean people eating together in a garden.

Switch the TV off and enjoy your meal. Monitor what the kids are eating. If you live alone, invite a co-worker, neighbor, or friend. You can even invite someone and prepare meals together.

Laugh Often – Have you heard of the popular saying, "Laughter is the best medicine"? This is true in the Mediterranean culture. Many are individuals with a big personality. Their conversations are full of humor. They love to tell stories. Enjoy life and keep a positive attitude/

Live a Simple Life – Consider food, for example. You won't find them buying too much of anything. The idea of buying any ingredient in bulk is foreign to them. They buy fresh, focusing on daily needs. And of course, fresh food is always best.

Enjoy Every Bite – Slow down and enjoy each bite. Many will eat for survival. But in the Mediterranean belt, they love their food. They enjoy it. Don't eat on the go. Sit down and have a proper meal.

Chapter 5

Health Benefits of the Mediterranean Diet

The Mediterranean diet is a valid ally for the protection of everyone 's health, as, based on vegetables, cereals, and extra virgin olive oil, it is able to bring to the body all those who are the fundamental substances for its proper operation. In this section of the book, we will share how it works and benefits to man.

How the Mediterranean diet works

The Mediterranean diet acts at various levels.

It reduces arterial hypertension, reduces bad LDL cholesterol, and increases good HDL cholesterol. It prevents and cures overweight and obesity. It helps prevent or better control type 2 diabetes.

It represents a factor that protects or stops the progression of atherosclerosis.

These benefits can be considered a real medicine both in those who only have these risk factors and in those who have already developed a heart attack.

Several components of the diet appear to have important beneficial effects.

The fish, especially the blue one, is rich in omega-3 and polyunsaturated fatty acids, which slow down the formation of atherosclerotic plaque, the first step for heart attack.

The extra-virgin olive oil, walnuts, and almonds give a good supply of the fundamental substances for the correct functioning of the body (carbohydrates, proteins, and fats) and are rich in micronutrients that have anti-atherosclerosis activity. They also reduce other risk factors for heart attack, such as high blood pressure. They improve insulin sensitivity, reducing the risk of type 2 diabetes.

The red wine is known that moderate amounts of wine promote good heart function as it is rich in resveratrol, a substance with important antioxidant activity.

Vitamin deficiency

One of the most important characteristics of the Mediterranean diet seems to be a correct balance between macro and micronutrients. Among the micronutrients, vitamins are essential for the body's well-being. The Mediterranean diet guarantees an adequate intake of both hydro and fat-soluble vitamins with great benefits.

The Mediterranean diet is rich in many important vitamins.

- *A: they are the precursors of retinol, an essential vitamin for the eyesight, the glands, and the immune system. The Mediterranean diet guarantees adequate income in more than 90% of the population because it is rich in vegetables and fish.*
- *B: the B vitamins are water-soluble and intervene in cellular metabolism. They are abundant in cereals and white meats, essential components of the Mediterranean diet.*
- *C: important for repairing vessels and has an antioxidant effect. The Mediterranean diet guarantees an adequate intake of this vitamin, being rich in fruit (in particular citrus fruits) and vegetables (in particular tomatoes).*
- *D: Adequate intake is essential for bone health. The Mediterranean diet, abundant in fish, guarantees an optimal supply of this vitamin.*
- *E: has antioxidant and anti-aging properties. It is abundantly contained in wheat, corn, rice, and green legumes.*
- *K: has an antihemorrhagic and osteoporosis action. It is contained in abundance in green legumes, in particular, the cruciferous (broccoli, cabbage).*
- *Folic acid: essential for the prevention of anemias, and in cellular metabolism, they are contained in large quantities in vegetables, in particular in broad-leaved ones.*

Cardiovascular disease and risk factors

Numerous studies have highlighted the important benefits of the Mediterranean diet on cardiovascular diseases. Not only on the main risk factors for these pathologies but also on the course of the disease once it occurs.

Oxidative stress and free radicals

Furthermore, all the components of the Mediterranean diet have high quantities of polyphenols, antioxidant substances, which counteract the action of free radicals and oxidative stress.

It involves the intake of high quantities of fruit and vegetables, rich in fiber. That limits the intestinal absorption of fats and slowdown that of sugars, thus preventing glycemic peaks.

Limit your intake of foods high in saturated fat such as red meats, cheeses, and sausages. Responsible, if in excess, for high cholesterol levels and, therefore, atherosclerotic risk.

Use aromatic herbs, which allow you to reduce your salt intake, thus helping to regulate blood pressure.

It is moderately low in calories, rich in fibers that increase the sense of satiety, and modulate the absorption of the various nutrients, favoring the control of body weight.

The metabolic syndrome

The set of risk factors mentioned above occurs in metabolic syndrome.

The Mediterranean diet is an important ally against this condition. Which exposes a subject to high cardiovascular risk.

Second type diabetes

A study presented by researchers reveals a new mechanism by which the Mediterranean diet could protect the vessels of people with type 2 diabetes.

The research was conducted on 215 subjects with newly diagnosed type 2 diabetes. These patients were divided into two groups. The first group was recommended a Mediterranean-type diet, the second group a non-Mediterranean low-fat diet.

At the end of the study, subjects who had followed the Mediterranean diet had significantly more endothelial progenitor cells than the other group.

Endothelial progenitor cells are young endothelial cells. That is, of the inside of the blood vessels. These cells have the function of repairing blood vessels when they are affected by ischemic damage.

It is the first diet-based study to demonstrate a beneficial effect of the Mediterranean diet on the regenerative capacity of the endothelium in a population of patients with newly diagnosed type 2 diabetes.

The study shows for the first time that following a Mediterranean diet is associated with the increase in circulating levels of endothelial cell progenitors.

These were important results, especially for patients with newly diagnosed type 2 diabetes, who were first advised to change their lifestyle with diet and structured physical activity, even before starting medical therapy.

Beneficial effects on tumors

Numerous studies have shown that the Mediterranean diet is able to reduce the risk of getting cancer.

A Mediterranean-type diet could prevent about:

- 25% of colorectal cancers
- 15-20% of breast cancers
- 10-15% of carcinomas of the prostate, endometrium, and pancreas

In fact, the Mediterranean diet has a high content of unsaturated fats, fibers, vitamins, and polyphenols, with an anti-free radical, anti-inflammatory, and antioxidant action.

Legumes contain phytoestrogens that modulate the action of sex hormones, hindering the growth of some of the most common tumors in the elderly population.

Fresh fruits and vegetables: rich in antioxidants capable of neutralizing free radicals, responsible for cellular degeneration. Vegetable fibers also regulate and improve intestinal function, freeing the body of toxins.

The fish, in particular, the blue one, is rich in omega-3 polyunsaturated fatty acids, coenzyme Q10, and selenium, antioxidant substances capable of counteracting the proliferation of cancer cells.

Extra virgin olive oil is rich in monounsaturated fatty acids, polyphenols, and vitamin E, which protect cell membranes from oxidative damage caused by free radicals.

Mediterranean diet allied to the brain

The Mediterranean diet is also the best food style to preserve our brain's decay.

In January 2017, a study from the University of Edinburgh published in the journal Neurology focused on brain size. The elderly who constantly follow this type of diet would have a less "consumed" brain than those who follow a different diet.

We know that as we age, the brain progressively loses neurons, the brain cells. This means reduced cognitive functions such as memory, learning ability, reasoning.

All the characteristics of the Mediterranean diet described above prevent the development of mild cognitive impairment and, therefore, of actual dementia.

Longevity and quality of life

An Italian study has recently shown that the Mediterranean diet improves the lifestyle of the elderly. The research was conducted by the Cnr Institute of Neuroscience and the University of Padua and published in the American Journal of Clinical Nutrition.

He highlighted how the Mediterranean diet ensures a lower prevalence of disability, depression, and pain in old age.

To reach this conclusion, the experts took into consideration 4,470 Americans with an average age of 61 years. Those who followed the Mediterranean diet have shown to have a higher quality of life, in particular, "a lower prevalence of disability and depression (about 30% less).

A diet that ensures longevity but also an excellent quality of life gained.

Chapter 6

Step by Step Instructions to Roll Out the Improvement

We are all involved in being lean, losing weight, getting a good diet plan, getting rid of cardiovascular and health-related illnesses. Typically, once you have a good diet plan such as the Mediterranean diet pan, the chances are that you will eventually reduce the number of calories in your body resulting in decreased heart-related issues.

The other benefits include weight shedding, fat burning and gradually slimming down. It is truly easy to implement diet plans like the Mediterranean diet plan. That's because you can't eat the gunk and bland vegetables that many people have to submit to just because they want to live longer and healthier.

You will enjoy delicious meals with the Mediterranean diet plan while still rising the chances of getting heart-related problems. Here are a few tips to help adopt the Mediterranean diet.

1. Decide on What Diet Type

Most of the people tend to worry about their diet plans consistently. They worry if it will work if they lose weight if they can reduce their chances of dying younger as a result of heart disease and cancer and, most importantly, worry if they can keep up with their diets. Okay, the thing is, if you really want to do this, you have to choose which choice you think works best for you.

There are two main dietary forms or regimens. You can do the form planned or the style Do-It-Yourself. It all depends on the makeup you have. For instance, some people don't like strict time tables and are more likely to fail to use them because they are instinctively opposed to things that make them feel like they're boxed in.

Though, other people find it exciting to chart a strategy and are more likely to stick to it. It all depends on the person that you are. So, whatever happens, just pick one out. If you don't know which group you're moving for, just go for one. You can always turn to the other, if you don't like it.

2. Find Recipes that Will Work for You

The taste of the people in the food is different. You need to find and stick to that which works for you. The basic components of the Mediterranean diet plan include, among others, olive oil, legumes, vegetables, nuts, grains, unprocessed carbohydrates, fish, reduced red meat consumption and saturated fat.

Now, if you just like eating them like that, then it's all right. But if you want to make it much more fun, you'd have to find recipes that work. The South Beach Diet recipes, for example, are great and fun to cook. So, find recipes that inculcate these and which are based on the Mediterranean diet.

3. Get Creative With the Diet

Since following a few diet plans, the reason many people return to eating junk is that the diets are either dull, repetitive or lacking in flavor. So, what you should do is just go for those delicious meals. Get yourself creative with the recipes. Try something new, and something different. Chances are if you're looking well enough, you'll find lots of Mediterranean diet recipes that will last you for a whole year and more.

4. Be Disciplined

Because the Mediterranean diet is really simple to use and apply, it is hardly called a diet by some. I just see it as an alternative lifestyle and food choices that help you stay healthy and live longer. The secret, then, is discipline. Stay focused and who knows, you could just give yourself an extra 15 years of health and life.

Chapter 7

A Delicious Path to Weight Loss

If you have attempted a lot of diets in the past, you will realize it can be a challenge finding a diet that is multi-faceted. This means that looking for a diet that will achieve weight loss, as well as keep you in optimum health, is difficult. Through this book so far, you have been able to learn a lot more about the Mediterranean diet, and you will realize it serves more than just one purpose. This makes it fairly obvious why many people from across the globe are now adopting the diet.

Some of the most outstanding reasons it is to become people's favorite diet plan include the fact it has been shown to improve the quality of life in terms of health status. In the countries where the diet originated, people seem to have a longer lifespan, and it is also a very effective diet to follow if you wish to cut down on unnecessary weight or simply correct your body figure. It is not a diet of deprivation; rather, it is a diet of moderation. It illustrates that making the right decisions, concerning what you eat, can uplift your life dramatically.

If your reason for adopting the Mediterranean diet is to get more insight on how you can shed weight and learn to stick to a regime that works, make sure you pay special attention to this section. Weight loss and one's outlook are matters that are dear to many people, and that is why people need to continue to learn that the Mediterranean diet plan is not a quick-fix to weight issue, neither is it a tedious, mundane regime that you have to bore yourself to death with. It is about considering a change in your lifestyle that will increase your happiness in leaps and bounds, especially how you feel about your physical body. Here are a few guidelines, which if properly adhered, will make the journey to adopting the Mediterranean diet fun and worthwhile.

The Mediterranean Diet is a series of health choices

It simply means you have to constantly and consciously choose good foods over the bad ones that are otherwise referred to as fast food and rich man's foods, like the burgers and other highly processed chemically-made foods. Although many people may argue they may not be aware that certain foods are unhealthy, they do not make a valid argument. You need to take a commonsensical approach to your food. Is it in its natural form? How has it been prepared? Does it contain a significant amount of added sugar? Have others labelled it as unhealthy? It is time to make the right choices.

The most important task for you as you make this healthy choice is to take a careful note of what the diet comprises, and each day choose to have a combination of three of the ingredients from those that make up the Mediterranean Diet that form a balanced diet. Other choices you have to make, in addition to choosing healthy foods, is the decision to control your calorie intake by managing your intake portions day by day. The easiest way to do this is to choose a smaller plate. By doing so, you will immediately begin to eat smaller portions, but you can still fill your plate the same way as if you were eating from a larger one.

Paying attention to lifestyle changes

The Mediterranean diet does not just focus on the food you eat, but also, to a large extent, how you live your life. You must have read by now about the history of the diet. Those from the Mediterranean origin, who strictly observed this diet, understood the importance of family and friends, and this is why meal times were revered in high regard. It is during these meal times that people would share their life experiences, and it was believed this sharing helped the participants deal with any stressful situation they might have been going through. What this is driving at is, the Mediterranean diet and stress do not mix. It is a diet that advocates you to have an excellent mental state, just as much as to fix yourself physically, inside and out.

One of the other areas to which you have to pay attention is the portions of food you consume. If you carefully study the diet, you will realize it entails some good proportion of carbohydrates and proteins, which, if not consumed in moderation, can have the effect of making you add weight, contrary to your expectation. The other component of the diet that you have to use in moderation is wine. It forms an integral part of the Mediterranean diet, but this does not in any way give you the leeway to overindulge in alcohol. Remember that the more wine you take, the more food you tend to eat, because wine has the effect of speeding up digestion.

Exercise is important

Even the people of old will tell you that all work with no play makes Jack a dull boy. In relation to the Mediterranean diet, if you work on getting your food portions and component right, but do not engage in physical activity to help your body assimilate the food properly, then you might as well forget about your weight loss goals. Slow down your fast-paced lifestyle and simply take the time to smell the flowers and to enjoy nature as you take a walk in the park or enjoy some swimming sessions.

Almost all diets mention the component of exercise is important, but on this diet, it is essential. You must exercise each day, whether it is light exercise or something intense that really gets your blood flowing. If possible, exercise with a loved one so you can share the experience and have just as much of an effect on your mind as you would on your body.

Set realistic goals

Do not just set the goals; stick to them. You definitely do not want to come up with goals you cannot realize and then blame it on the diet and conclude that it does not work. For example, even if you were consuming just the food components in the Mediterranean diet pyramid, but heaping your plate with excess amounts and doing no exercise, it would definitely not be the diet's fault that you added more weight instead of losing. However, if you consider taking in low-calorie foods in large quantities and more frequently, for example fruits and vegetables, you are good to go. This may seem like straightforward and logical reasoning, but when it comes to issues of body weight, many people become unreasonable and make every possible excuse they can. Eat right, exercise, and you will most assuredly, lose your excess weight.

Say no to food cravings

Do you know why people tend to find it very challenging to realize their goal of losing weight within a specified time? It is the little devil called craving. It is true that cravings could be a result of physiological or psychological factors or a combination of both, but they need to be dealt with accordingly. What do you do when you feel the urge to snack on sweet things, like chocolate? It is likely that you reach out for them and take in 'just a little bit'. Usually, what would happen is you start small, and ten minutes later, you are staring at an empty wrapper with a guilty look on your face.

Change this destructive behavior as you choose this wholesome diet. Choose to take a cup of water or yogurt instead. Other suggestions for dealing with cravings are ensuring you do not skip meals, as this only makes the craving worse. The result of this is binge eating, or eating the foods that are wrong for you in excess. You should also ensure that you eat more proteins, such as fish, a little often as this will slow down digestion a bit, hence, reducing chances of a full-blown chocolate craving. The right foods will fill you up and balance your body, so sugar and carb cravings are kept at bay.

Fruits, vegetables, and nuts, if incorporated during a meal, will keep away the urge to snack on sweet bites every now and then. They are rich in fiber and the right fats, and they contain sugar in its natural form.

Quit diets once and for all

With all the information available in the various diets you can try in order to lose weight, you are bound to get confused and especially so if you try to work on them as you observe the Mediterranean diet regime. You must have read about those diets that advise you to keep off carbohydrates and proteins and purely cut down to fruits and vegetables only.

There are also diets that insist you should live on soup and health shakes for a long period. Or even some that cut down your intake of certain food groups completely. What such diets don't point out is that you need carbohydrates to energize your body and proteins to build the body. This is the reason most of these diets do not work for long, because at some point, low energy and blood sugar level will dictate that you eat heavy foods. As long as the body receives what it requires in the right quantities, it will balance itself and lead you to a healthy weight. The moment you abuse your body by making the wrong food choices, some of which border on the extreme, the easier it becomes to fall off the wagon on fad diets.

Do away with stress

Stress is controllable; it is just a matter of how you choose to respond to stressors and factors that trigger you to become unhappy. Learn how to manage your stress factors in simple ways, like getting enough sleep, meditating, exercising, and deep breathing and walking away from stressful situations, it is possible. Practice this and watch as the Mediterranean diet transforms you into the person you want to be. Another way this diet helps you relieve the stresses you face each day is the focus on family and relationships, sharing meals, and experiences. When you have someone to share with, what could have appeared as a large issue, is brought back down to size.

Chapter 8

Essential Mediterranean Food

The principle behind Mediterranean dishes is natural, simple ingredients that can be found on the coast region. This leads to a variety of vegetables, fruit, whole grains, beans, healthy fats, red wine, beef, and fish. It's considered one of the healthiest diets.

Fruits & Vegetables

The first part of the Mediterranean diet is fresh fruits and vegetables. Most vegetables and fruits are low in fat and high in fiber, which make them heart healthy. They can help with weight loss too.

They're also full of antioxidants which can help to reduce inflammation and slow down the aging process.

The antioxidants include vitamins A, vitamin C, vitamin E and vitamin K. they can help to remove harmful free radicals that can cause the oxidation of LDL, also known as bad cholesterol.

Whole Grains

This is also a must for the Mediterranean diet. Refined grains have been stripped of nutrients during the refinement process, which means they aren't as healthy as whole grains which have more nutrition. Whole grains have bran, endosperm and germ which are great for your health.

Some whole grain examples are brown rice, barley, bulgur, millet, oat, rye, teff, and wheat. Whole grains have quite a few benefits as well since they are more satisfying to your hunger and have phytochemicals which are disease-fighting chemicals.

Using Olive Oil

Olive oil has a lot of monounsaturated fats which can protect against heart disease because it keeps LDL levels, bad cholesterol, low and HDL levels, good cholesterol, high. Most Mediterranean meals are prepared by liberally using olive oil. Also, on the Mediterranean diet most foods are grilled or baked, which is easier to do with olive oil.

Fish & Chicken

The Mediterranean diet often includes and abundance of fresh fish because of the proximity of the area to the sea. Fish has a lot of omega-3 fatty acids which have various heart healthy benefits including reducing triglycerides, inflammation and even cholesterol. There are various types of fish to choose from as well, including salmon, mackerel, herring, sardines, trout and albacore tuna. Chicken can also be used in place of fish to replace red meat. It isn't as healthy as fish, but it does have lower saturated fats and cholesterol than red meat.

Nuts

Unsalted nuts are often eaten as a snack in Mediterranean countries. However, the US is more likely to go for things such as crackers or potato chips which have no health benefits. Nuts can also be included in desserts and savory dishes. Pine nuts can be used to make homemade pesto, and you'll find walnuts are often in bread dough. Nuts are a wonderful source of monounsaturated fat, and they're packed full of protein and fiber. They can also contain various minerals and vitamins which will help to improve your overall health.

Red Wine

Small amounts of alcohol is consumed with most meals, especially red wine, in Mediterranean countries. It's been proven that alcoholic drinks, such as red wine, have healthy heart benefits. Red wine has an antioxidant called flavonoids which can prevent fatty deposits from building up in the artery walls. Even the American Heart Association recommends one to two drinks a day for men and women. These drinks are only suppose to be four ounces each.

Spices

There are many spices and herbs that are used in the Mediterranean diet that also provide health benefits, including garlic. While these herbs and spices help to make the food taste great, their benefits to your health is the real magic.

The most common herbs and spices in this area are garlic, anise, basil, bay leaf, fennel, lavender, cumin, mint, marjoram, oregano, pepper, rosemary, sumaci, parsley, thyme and tarragon. Cutting down on salt can help to lower blood pressure, which is also a risk for heart disease, and these flavors help to lower your intake of salt. Garlic is a great way to spice up your meal, and you may not even know that the salt is missing!

Dairy

Full fat dairy products, including cheese and whole milk, are eaten in small amounts in Mediterranean countries. This helps to keep the saturated fat intake down. However, traditional cheeses such as goat cheese and feta cheese are lower in fat than hard cheeses such as Cheddar, which is extremely popular in the US. There is also yogurt which is eaten more frequently by being included in various dishes and desserts which is very healthy. Eggs can also be eaten regularly, but egg yolk is limited in this diet. Egg yolk should be limited to four per week to help to control your saturated fat intake. Though, egg whites can be eaten much more often.

Legumes

The importance of legumes is also emphasized in the Mediterranean diet. These include beans, peas, lentils and snap peas. Legumes have a high fiber and protein count which is a great addition to your diet.

Foods to Avoid

You should reduce red meat in the Mediterranean diet since it can contribute to heart disease, but you don't have to completely avoid it. With this diet, you don't have to completely avoid anything, but there are certain items that should be reduced and eaten sparingly. When you want to eat something like red meat, try to choose a small portion of lean red meat instead, and keep it down to three to four times per month. Here are some more foods to limit or avoid all together if possible.

Added Sugars: This includes candies, ice cream, table sugar and soda.

Refined Grains: This includes pasta that's made of refined wheat and white bread.

Trans Fat: This can be found in various processed foods, but it's also in margarine!

Refined Oils: This includes cottonseed oil, vegetable oil, canola oil and soybean oil.

- *Processed Meats:* Some common examples are processed hot dogs and sausages.
- *Highly Processed Foods:* This includes anything that is labeled "diet", "low fat" or was obviously made in a factory. Remember that you should be concentrating on whole, natural ingredients.

Swapping Food Out

If you're trying to stick to a Mediterranean diet, you need to know what common food you're eating can be swapped with to help keep you on track.

- *Butter:* Just swap it out for olive oil.
- *Salt:* Just swap it out for a variety of herbs and spices instead.
- *Mayonnaise:* Mayonnaise can be swapped out for mashed avocado.
- *Beer:* It's better to switch to a glass or two of red wine which has heart benefits.
- *Beef:* Beef isn't great for you, but you can usually swap it out for salmon which can easily be found at most grocery stores.
- *Potato Chips:* Instead of munching on something that has no health benefits, choose a bag of mixed nuts. Just make sure they're unsalted.
- *Jam or Jelly:* Swap it out for fresh fruit instead. You may want to even puree it in a food processor.
- *Rice or Bread:* While you can eat whole wheat bread and some rice on the Mediterranean diet, cut it back. If you're trying to cut back try to switch for legumes instead.
- *Cakes & Cookies:* Try vegetables and hummus for a healthy alternative that will curb your appetite.

The Take Away

Now that you know what you should and shouldn't eat, you need to make sure that you avoid as much temptation as possible. Clean out your home from things that are too unhealthy, especially at the beginning of your dietary change. It can be hard to stick to a lifestyle change. You'll also need to keep in mind your portion control, and you'll need to start making some time for physical activity even if it's just twenty minutes a day.

Chapter 9

Planning Your Mediterranean Diet

Proper preparation guarantees success at the end. Deciding to follow the Mediterranean diet program will not help you if there are internal flaws. If you have access to a dietician, then consult with him/her. The expert will chart out a watertight food plan that will give you the gifts of health and physical wellbeing. Thanks to food magazines, online articles, and blogs, even a beginner will be able to identify the critical points of the Mediterranean Diet.

A proportionate combination of elements

A novice may think that the Mediterranean diet is all about munching on green salads, with olive oil dressing and taking sips of red wine. Though there is a difference between the western and the European cooking styles, these people understand the importance of a balanced meal. Your body needs carbohydrates, fats, proteins, roughage, and minerals to stay in top shape. Absence of any of these nutritional elements will make you internally weak.

A close look at the Mediterranean Diet pyramid ensures that every meal you have contains all elements in a balanced proportion. If you are not good with numbers and measurements, the simplest way is to divide the plate into three parts. Fill half of it with fruits and veggies, while one-quarter will be composed of assorted whole grains. The remaining one-quarter will contain lean meat, especially fish.

Understand the importance of whole products

No Mediterranean household invests money in processed foods. Processed foods are chemically treated in the factories to enhance their appearance. In the process, the nutritional value gets depleted drastically. The Mediterranean diet stresses the use of whole products, like vegetables, nuts, legumes, nuts, and whole grains.

Elements to be considered by Mediterranean Diet enthusiasts

Binge on veggies – The key feature of this diet is fresh fruits and vegetables. People in the Mediterranean areas depend on fresh farm products only. This diet plan consists of anything between seven and ten fruit-veggies servings on a daily basis. The high percentage of veggies and fruits will put a stopper on heart-related ailments. You don't have to sit with a bowl of vegetables and assorted fruit mixtures every time you feel hungry. Simply adding some spinach to your morning omelet or loading avocados onto your evening sandwich will do the trick. Apple slices, with nuts, will substitute for an unhealthy burger.

Replace meat with fresh fish – Lack of protein in the diet will impair the development of our muscles. In the Mediterranean diet, people stress eating fatty fish instead of red meat. Too much consumption of red meat will pave the path for high BP and heart diseases.

To attain protein, you will have to depend on fish like mackerel, salmon, herring, and tuna. Apart from being protein-rich, these are also potential sources of Omega-3 fatty acids. It will keep any inflammation under check and will also boost up the good cholesterol levels. Shellfish are also included in this diet plan. These are considered functional lean proteins. Additionally, turkey meat, chicken, and eggs are common ingredients in Mediterranean dishes.

Swap processed butter with olive oil – While most other diet plans stress the core ingredients, the cooking medium is also considered necessary in the Mediterranean diet. The type of fat obtained from olive oil will not create a negative impact on the cardiovascular system. Additionally, it will also come in handy to help manage body weight.

Go for healthy dairy products – A dollop of cheese has the power to enhance the flavor of any dish. But processed cheese will harm the heart and increase body fat drastically. Thus, the Mediterranean diet supplements this with natural dairy products. Naturally manufactured flavored cheeses, for instance, Parmesan or feta will intensify the flavors sans the adverse effects. Fermented or plain Greek yogurts are also standard on this diet list. Consuming such milk products makes it easy for the body to break them down and allows for better absorption.

Pick whole grains – Whole grains are another essential part of the Mediterranean diet. If you think that munching on unprocessed nuts will increase your body weight, then it is time to shun the thought forever.

Most types of nuts used in this diet program contain healthy fats. Other whole cereals will ensure that blood sugar, blood pressure, cholesterol and sugar levels stay within the normal ranges. Consuming unprocessed whole grains will increase Vitamin B and other fiber-based components in your body. Additionally, this fiber will also act as roughage that will ease your gut and intestinal functions.

Limit sugar intakes – Skipping sugar entirely will cause the average blood sugar level to fall. But the Mediterranean diet highlights the use of natural sugar supplements like pure honey instead of processed white sugar granules. It is best to keep its use within healthy limits. Unprocessed brown sugar is also used in Mediterranean dishes to add some sweetness.

Healthy snacking ideas – The lazy afternoons and the evenings are the perfect time for some snacks. While an average American will opt for a pizza or burger, people following the Mediterranean diet will go for an assortment of nuts and crunchy fruits. The nut-n-fruit salad, with proper dressing, will not only meet your hunger, but will add nutritional value as well.

Importance of red wine – The importance of red wine has been documented since time immemorial. The Mediterranean climate offers the ideal condition for the growth of several types of grapes. A glass of red wine is an inseparable part of any Mediterranean meal. Red wine is good for heart, blood circulation, kidney, stomach, and skin. Two glasses of wine with lunch and dinner will make your Mediterranean diet complete.

Chapter 10

21-Day Meal Plan

Day	Breakfast	Lunch	Dinner	Snack/Dessert
1	Breakfast Egg On Avocado	Italian Lamb Shanks	Stuffed Sardines	Mediterranean Flatbread With Toppings
2	Breakfast Egg-Artichoke Casserole	Beef Goulash	Mini Greek Meatloaves	Smoked Salmon And Goat Cheese Bites
3	Brekky Egg-Potato Hash	Instant Pot Korean Beef	Yogurt-And-Herb-Marinated Pork Tenderloin	Mediterranean Chickpea Bowl
4	Dill And Tomato Frittata	Beef Ragu	Rosemary Potatoes	Hummus Snack Bowl
5	Paleo Almond Banana Pancakes	Sloppy Joe With Beef	Delicious Italian Bell Pepper	Crock-Pot Paleo Chunky Mix
6	Banana-Coconut Breakfast	Beef & Tomato Soup	Pesto Zucchini	Smoked Eggplant Dip

7	Basil And Tomato Soup	Ground Lamb Curry	Pesto Cauliflower	Pumpkin Cream
8	Butternut Squash Hummus	Rosemary Lamb	Italian Tomato Mushrooms	Italian Oven Roasted Vegetables
9	Cajun Jambalaya Soup	Thyme Lamb	Chickpea & Potato	Greek Spinach Yogurt Artichoke Dip
10	Collard Green Wrap Greek Style	Garlic Lamb Shanks With Port	Zesty Green Beans	Sautéed Apricots
11	Portobello Mushroom Pizza	Sea Bass In A Pan With Peppers	Walnut-Rosemary Crusted Salmon	Spiced Kale Chips
12	Roasted Root Veggies	Crusty Tuna Patties	Caprese Stuffed Portobello Mushrooms	Yogurt Dip
13	Amazingly Good Parsley Tabbouleh	Baked Teriyaki Salmon	Greek Salad Nachos	Zucchini Fritters
14	Appetizing Mushroom Lasagna	Whole Roasted Mackerel	Greek Chicken With Lemon Vinaigrette	Chia And Berries Smoothie Bowl

			And Roasted Spring Vegetables	
15	Artichokes, Olives & Tuna Pasta	White Fish Sautéed With Lemon, Capers And Herbs	Chicken In Tomato-Balsamic Pan Sauce	Cucumber Bites
16	Baked Ricotta With Pears	Baked Fish With Olives, Tomatoes, And Eggplant	Chicken Souvlaki Kebabs With Mediterranean Couscous	Stuffed Avocado
17	Mediterranean Fruit Bulgur Breakfast Bowl	Grilled White Fish With Fresh Basil Pesto	Caprese Chicken Hasselback Style	Wrapped Plums
18	Scrambled Eggs With Goat Cheese And Roasted Peppers	White Fish With Chickpeas And Chorizo	Simple Grilled Salmon With Veggies	Cucumber Sandwich Bites
19	Marinara Eggs With Parsley	Fresh Salmon With Lemon Butter And	Greek Turkey Burgers With	Cucumber Rolls

		New Potatoes	Spinach, Feta &Tzatziki	
20	Italian Breakfast Bruschetta	Fresh Fish Puttanesca Salad With Couscous	Mediterranean Chicken Quinoa Bowl	Olives And Cheese Stuffed Tomatoes
21	Julene's Green Juice	Tuna Croquettes	Creamy Dill Potatoes	Crème Caramel

Chapter 11

Breakfast & Brunch Recipes

Breakfast Egg on Avocado

Preparation Time: 10 minutes | Cooking Time: 15 minutes | Servings: 6

Ingredients:

1 tsp garlic powder

1/2 tsp sea salt

1/4 cup Parmesan cheese (grated or shredded)

1/4 tsp black pepper

3 medium avocados (cut in half, pitted, skin on)

6 medium eggs

Directions:

Prepare muffin tins and preheat the oven to 350oF. To ensure that the egg would fit inside the cavity of the avocado, lightly scrape off 1/3 of the meat. Place avocado on muffin tin to ensure that it faces with the top up. Evenly season each avocado with pepper, salt, and garlic powder. Add one egg on each avocado cavity and garnish tops with cheese. Pop in the oven and bake until the egg white is set, about 15 minutes. Serve and enjoy.

Nutrition: Calories: 252 Protein: 14.0g Carbs: 4.0g Fat: 20.0g

Breakfast Egg-artichoke Casserole

Preparation Time: 8 minutes | Cooking Time: 35 minutes | Servings: 8

Ingredients:

16 large eggs

14 ounce can artichoke hearts, drained

10-ounce box frozen chopped spinach, thawed and drained well

1 cup shredded white cheddar

1 garlic clove, minced

1 teaspoon salt

1/2 cup parmesan cheese

1/2 cup ricotta cheese

1/2 teaspoon dried thyme

1/2 teaspoon crushed red pepper

1/4 cup milk

1/4 cup shaved onion

Directions:

Lightly grease a 9x13-inch baking dish with cooking spray and preheat the oven to 350oF.

In a large mixing bowl, add eggs and milk. Mix thoroughly.

With a paper towel, squeeze out the excess moisture from the spinach leaves and add to the bowl of eggs.

Into small pieces, break the artichoke hearts and separate the leaves. Add to the bowl of eggs.

Except for the ricotta cheese, add remaining ingredients in the bowl of eggs and mix thoroughly.

Pour egg mixture into the prepared dish.

Evenly add dollops of ricotta cheese on top of the eggs and then pop in the oven.

Bake until eggs are set and doesn't jiggle when shook, about 35 minutes.

Remove from the oven and evenly divide into suggested servings. Enjoy.

Nutrition:

Calories: 302, Protein: 22.6g, Carbs: 10.8g, Fat: 18.7g

Brekky Egg-potato Hash

Preparation Time: 5 minutes | Cooking Time: 25 minutes | Servings: 2

Ingredients:

1 zucchini, diced

1/2 cup chicken broth

½ pound cooked chicken

1 tablespoon olive oil

4 ounces shrimp

Salt and ground black pepper to taste

1 large sweet potato, diced

2 eggs

1/4 teaspoon cayenne pepper

2 teaspoons garlic powder

1 cup fresh spinach (optional)

Directions:

In a skillet, add the olive oil.

Fry the shrimp, cooked chicken and sweet potato for 2 minutes.

Add the cayenne pepper, garlic powder and salt, and toss for 4 minutes.

Add the zucchini and toss for another 3 minutes.

Whisk the eggs in a bowl and add to the skillet.

Season using salt and pepper. Cover with the lid.

Cook for 1 minute and add the chicken broth.

Cover and cook for another 8 minutes on high heat.

Add the spinach and toss for 2 more minutes.

Serve immediately.

Nutrition:

Calories: 190, Protein: 11.7g, Carbs: 2.9g, Fat: 12.3g

Dill and Tomato Frittata

Preparation Time: 10 minutes | Cooking Time: 35 minutes | Servings: 6

Ingredients:

Pepper and salt to taste

1 tsp red pepper flakes

2 garlic cloves, minced

½ cup crumbled goat cheese – optional

2 tbsp fresh chives, chopped

2 tbsp fresh dill, chopped

4 tomatoes, diced

8 eggs, whisked

1 tsp coconut oil

Directions:

Grease a 9-inch round baking pan and preheat oven to 325oF.

In a large bowl, mix well all ingredients and pour into prepped pan.

Pop into the oven and bake until middle is cooked through around 30-35 minutes.

Remove from oven and garnish with more chives and dill.

Nutrition:

Calories: 149, Protein: 13.26g, Carbs: 9.93g, Fat: 10.28g

Paleo Almond Banana Pancakes

Preparation Time: 10 minutes | Cooking Time: 10 minutes | Servings: 3

Ingredients:

¼ cup almond flour

½ teaspoon ground cinnamon

3 eggs

1 banana, mashed

1 tablespoon almond butter

1 teaspoon vanilla extract

1 teaspoon olive oil

Sliced banana to serve

Directions:

Whisk the eggs in a mixing bowl until they become fluffy.

In another bowl, mash the banana using a fork and add to the egg mixture.

Add the vanilla, almond butter, cinnamon and almond flour.

Mix into a smooth batter.

Heat the olive oil in a skillet.

Add one spoonful of the batter and fry them on both sides.

Keep doing these steps until you are done with all the batter.

Add some sliced banana on top before serving.

Nutrition:

Calories: 306, Protein: 14.4g, Carbs: 3.6g, Fat: 26.0g

Banana-Coconut Breakfast

Preparation Time: 10 minutes | Cooking Time: 3 minutes | Servings: 4

Ingredients:

1 ripe banana

1 cup desiccated coconut

1 cup coconut milk

3 tablespoons raisins, chopped

2 tablespoon ground flax seed

1 teaspoon vanilla

A dash of cinnamon

A dash of nutmeg

Salt to taste

Directions:

Place all ingredients in a deep pan.

Allow to simmer for 3 minutes on low heat.

Place in individual containers.

Put a label and store in the fridge.

Allow to thaw at room temperature before heating in the microwave oven.

Nutrition:

Calories:279, Carbs: 25.46g, Protein: 6.4g, Fat: g, Fiber: 5.9g

Basil and Tomato Soup

Preparation Time: 10 minutes | Cooking Time: 25 minutes | Servings: 2

Ingredients:

Salt and pepper to taste

2 bay leaves

1 ½ cups almond milk, unsweetened

½ tsp raw apple cider vinegar

1/3 cup basil leaves

¼ cup tomato paste

3 cups tomatoes, chopped

1 medium celery stalk, chopped

1 medium carrot, chopped

1 medium garlic clove, minced

½ cup white onion

2 tbsp vegetable broth

Directions:

Heat the vegetable broth in a large saucepan over medium heat.

Add the onions and cook for 3 minutes. Add the garlic and cook for another minute.

Add the celery and carrots and cook for 1 minute.

Mix in the tomatoes and bring to a boil. Simmer for 15 minutes.

Add the almond milk, basil and bay leaves. Season with salt and pepper to taste.

Nutrition:

Calories: 213, Carbs: 42.0g, Protein: 6.9g, Fat: 3.9g

Butternut Squash Hummus

Preparation Time: 10 minutes | Cooking Time: 15 minutes | Servings: 8 |

Ingredients:

2 pounds butternut squash, seeded and peeled

1 tablespoon olive oil

¼ cup tahini

2 tablespoons lemon juice

2 cloves of garlic, minced

Salt and pepper to taste

Directions:

Heat the oven to 3000F.

Coat the butternut squash with olive oil.

Place in a baking dish and bake for 15 minutes in the oven.

Once the squash is cooked, place in a food processor together with the rest of the ingredients.

Pulse until smooth.

Place in individual containers.

Put a label and store in the fridge.

Allow to warm at room temperature before heating in the microwave oven.

Serve with carrots or celery sticks.

Nutrition:

Calories: 115, Carbs: 15.8g, Protein: 2.5g, Fat:5.8g, Fiber: 6.7g

Cajun Jambalaya Soup

Preparation Time: 10 minutes | Cooking Time: 6 hours | Servings: 6

Ingredients:

¼ cup Frank's red hot sauce

3 tbsp Cajun seasoning

2 cups okra

½ head of cauliflower

1 pkg spicy Andouille sausages

4 oz chicken, diced

1 lb. large shrimps, raw and deveined

2 bay leaves

2 cloves garlic, diced

1 large can organic diced tomatoes

1 large onion, chopped

4 pepper

5 cups chicken stock

Directions:

In slow cooker, place the bay leaves, red hot sauce, Cajun seasoning, chicken, garlic, onions, and peppers.

Set slow cooker on low and cook for 5 ½ hours.

Then add sausages cook for 10 minutes.

Meanwhile, pulse cauliflower in food processor to make cauliflower rice.

Add cauliflower rice into slow cooker. Cook for 20 minutes.

Serve and enjoy.

Nutrition:

Calories: 155, Carbs: 13.9g, Protein: 17.4g, Fat: 3.8g

Collard Green Wrap Greek Style

Preparation Time: 10 minutes | Cooking Time: 0 minutes | Servings: 4

Ingredients:

½ block feta, cut into 4 (1-inch thick) strips (4-oz)

½ cup purple onion, diced

½ medium red bell pepper, julienned

1 medium cucumber, julienned

4 large cherry tomatoes, halved

4 large collard green leaves, washed

8 whole kalamata olives, halved

1 cup full-fat plain Greek yogurt

1 tablespoon white vinegar

1 teaspoon garlic powder

2 tablespoons minced fresh dill

2 tablespoons olive oil

2.5-ounces cucumber, seeded and grated (¼-whole)

Salt and pepper to taste

Directions:

Make the Tzatziki sauce first: make sure to squeeze out all the excess liquid from the cucumber after grating. In a small bowl, mix all sauce ingredients thoroughly and refrigerate.

Prepare and slice all wrap ingredients.

On a flat surface, spread one collard green leaf. Spread 2 tablespoons of Tzatziki sauce on middle of the leaf.

Layer ¼ of each of the tomatoes, feta, olives, onion, pepper, and cucumber. Place them on the center of the leaf, like piling them high instead of spreading them.

Fold the leaf like you would a burrito. Repeat process for remaining ingredients.

Serve and enjoy.

Nutrition:

Calories: 165.3, Protein: 7.0g, Carbs: 9.9g, Fat: 11.2g

Portobello Mushroom Pizza

Preparation Time: 10 minutes | Cooking Time: 12 minutes | Servings: 4 |

Ingredients:

½ teaspoon red pepper flakes

A handful of fresh basil, chopped

1 can black olives, chopped

1 medium onion, chopped

1 green pepper, chopped

¼ cup chopped roasted yellow peppers

½ cup prepared nut cheese, shredded

2 cups prepared gluten-free pizza sauce

8 Portobello mushrooms, cleaned and stems removed

Directions:

Preheat the oven toaster.

Take a baking sheet and grease it. Set aside.

Place the Portobello mushroom cap-side down and spoon 2 tablespoon of packaged pizza sauce on the underside of each cap. Add nut cheese and top with the remaining ingredients.

Broil for 12 minutes or until the toppings are wilted.

Nutrition:

Calories: 578, Carbs: 73.0g, Protein: 24.4g, Fat: 22.4g

Roasted Root Veggies

Preparation Time: 10 minutes | Cooking Time: 1 hour and 30 minutes | Servings: 6

Ingredients:

2 tbsp olive oil

1 head garlic, cloves separated and peeled

1 large turnip, peeled and cut into ½-inch pieces

1 medium sized red onion, cut into ½-inch pieces

1 ½ lbs. beets, trimmed but not peeled, scrubbed and cut into ½-inch pieces

1 ½ lbs. Yukon gold potatoes, unpeeled, cut into ½-inch pieces

2 ½ lbs. butternut squash, peeled, seeded, cut into ½-inch pieces

Directions:

Grease 2 rimmed and large baking sheets. Preheat oven to 425oF. In a large bowl, mix all ingredients thoroughly. Into the two baking sheets, evenly divide the root vegetables, spread in one layer. Season generously with pepper and salt. Pop into the oven and roast for 1 hour and 15 minute or until golden brown and tender. Remove from oven and let it cool for at least 15 minutes before serving.

Nutrition: Calories: 298 Carbs: 61.1g Protein: 7.4g Fat: 5.0g

Amazingly Good Parsley Tabbouleh

Preparation Time: 10 minutes | Cooking Time: 15 minutes | Servings: 4 |

Ingredients:

¼ cup chopped fresh mint

¼ cup lemon juice

¼ tsp salt

½ cup bulgur

½ tsp minced garlic

1 cup water

1 small cucumber, peeled, seeded and diced

2 cups finely chopped flat-leaf parsley

2 tbsp extra virgin olive oil

2 tomatoes, diced

4 scallions, thinly sliced

Pepper to taste

Directions:

Cook bulgur according to package instructions. Drain and set aside to cool for at least 15 minutes.

In a small bowl, mix pepper, salt, garlic, oil, and lemon juice.

Transfer bulgur into a large salad bowl and mix in scallions, cucumber, tomatoes, mint, and parsley.

Pour in dressing and toss well to coat.

Place bowl in ref until chilled before serving.

Nutrition:

Calories: 134.8, Carbs: 13g, Protein: 7.2g, Fat: 6g

Appetizing Mushroom Lasagna

Preparation Time: 10 minutes | Cooking Time: 75 minutes | Servings: 8

Ingredients:

½ cup grated Parmigiano-Reggiano cheese

No boil lasagna noodles

Cooking spray

¼ cup all-purpose flour

3 cups reduced fat milk, divided

2 tbsp chopped fresh chives, divided

1/3 cup less fat cream cheese

½ cup white wine

6 garlic cloves, minced and divided

1 ½ tbsp. Chopped fresh thyme

½ tsp freshly ground black pepper, divided

1 tsp salt, divided

1 package 4 oz pre-sliced exotic mushroom blend

1 package 8oz pre-sliced cremini mushrooms

1 ¼ cups chopped shallots

2 tbsp olive oil, divided

1 tbsp butter

1 oz dried porcini mushrooms

1 cup boiling water

Directions:

For 30 minutes, submerge porcini in 1 cup boiling hot water. With a sieve, strain mushroom and reserve liquid.

Over medium high fire, melt butter on a fry pan. Mix in 2 tbsp oil and for three minutes fry shallots. Add ¼ tsp pepper, ½ tsp salt, exotic mushrooms and cremini, cook for six minutes. Stir in 3 garlic cloves and thyme, cook for a minute. Bring to a boil as you pour wine by increasing fire to high and cook until liquid evaporates around a minute. Turn off fire and stir in porcini mushrooms, 1 tbsp chives and cream cheese. Mix well.

On medium high fire, place a separate medium sized pan with 1 tbsp oil. Sauté for half a minute 3 garlic cloves. Then bring to a boil as you pour 2 ¾ cups milk and reserved porcini liquid. Season with remaining pepper and salt. In a separate bowl, whisk together flour and ¼ cup milk and pour into pan. Stir constantly and cook until mixture thickens.

In a greased rectangular glass dish, pour and spread ½ cup of sauce, top with lasagna, top with half of mushroom mixture and another layer of lasagna. Repeat the layering process and instead of lasagna layer, end with the mushroom mixture and cover with cheese.

For 45 minutes, bake the lasagna in a preheated 350oF oven. Garnish with chives before serving.

Nutrition:

Calories: 268, Carbs: 29.6g Protein: 10.2g Fat: 12.6g

Artichokes, Olives & Tuna Pasta

Preparation Time: 10 minutes | Cooking Time: 15 minutes | Servings: 4

Ingredients:

¼ cup chopped fresh basil

¼ cup chopped green olives

¼ tsp freshly ground pepper

½ cup white wine

½ tsp salt, divided

1 10-oz package frozen artichoke hearts, thawed and squeezed dry

2 cups grape tomatoes, halved

2 tbsp lemon juice

2 tsp chopped fresh rosemary

2 tsp freshly grated lemon zest

3 cloves garlic, minced

4 tbsp extra virgin olive oil, divided

6-oz whole wheat penne pasta

8-oz tuna steak, cut into 3 pieces

Directions:

Cook penne pasta according to package instructions. Drain and set aside.

Preheat grill to medium high.

In bowl, toss and mix ¼ tsp pepper, ¼ tsp salt, 1 tsp rosemary, lemon zest, 1 tbsp oil and tuna pieces.

Grill tuna for 3 minutes per side. Allow to cool and flake into bite sized pieces.

On medium fire, place a large nonstick saucepan and heat 3 tbsp oil.

Sauté remaining rosemary, garlic olives, and artichoke hearts for 4 minutes

Add wine and tomatoes, bring to a boil and cook for 3 minutes while stirring once in a while.

Add remaining salt, lemon juice, tuna pieces and pasta. Cook until heated through.

To serve, garnish with basil and enjoy.

Nutrition:

Calories: 127.6, Carbs: 13g, Protein: 7.2g, Fat: 5.2g

Baked Ricotta With Pears

Preparation Time: 5 minutes | Cooking Time: 25 minutes | Servings: 4

Ingredients:

Nonstick cooking spray

1 (16-ounce) container whole-milk ricotta cheese

2 large eggs

¼ cup white whole-wheat flour or whole-wheat pastry flour

1 tablespoon sugar

1 teaspoon vanilla extract

¼ teaspoon ground nutmeg

1 pear, cored and diced

2 tablespoons water

1 tablespoon honey

Directions:

Preheat the oven to 400°F. Spray four 6-ounce ramekins with nonstick cooking spray.

In a large bowl, beat together the ricotta, eggs, flour, sugar, vanilla, and nutmeg. Spoon into the ramekins. Bake for 22 to 25 minutes, or until the ricotta is just about set. Remove from the oven and cool slightly on racks.

While the ricotta is baking, in a small saucepan over medium heat, simmer the pear in the water for 10 minutes, until slightly softened. Remove from the heat, and stir in the honey.

Serve the ricotta ramekins topped with the warmed pear.

Nutrition:

Calories: 312

Total Fat: 17g

Saturated Fat: 10g

Cholesterol: 163mg

Sodium: 130mg

Total Carbohydrates: 23g

Fiber: 2g Protein: 17g

Mediterranean Fruit Bulgur Breakfast Bowl

Preparation Time: 5 minutes | Cooking Time: 15 minutes | Servings: 6

Ingredients:

1½ cups uncooked bulgur

2 cups 2% milk

1 cup water

½ teaspoon ground cinnamon

2 cups frozen (or fresh, pitted) dark sweet cherries

8 dried (or fresh) figs, chopped

½ cup chopped almonds

¼ cup loosely packed fresh mint, chopped

Warm 2% milk, for serving (optional)

Directions:

In a medium saucepan, combine the bulgur, milk, water, and cinnamon. Stir once, then bring just to a boil. Cover, reduce the heat to medium-low, and simmer for 10 minutes or until the liquid is absorbed.

Turn off the heat, but keep the pan on the stove, and stir in the frozen cherries (no need to thaw), figs, and almonds. Stir well, cover for 1 minute, and let the hot bulgur thaw the cherries and partially hydrate the figs. Stir in the mint.

Scoop into serving bowls. Serve with warm milk, if desired. You can also serve it chilled.

Nutrition:

Calories: 301, Total Fat: 6g, Saturated Fat: 1g, Cholesterol: 7mg, Sodium: 40mg, Total Carbohydrates: 57g, Fiber: 9g, Protein: 9g

Scrambled Eggs With Goat Cheese And Roasted Peppers

Preparation Time: 5 minutes | Cooking Time: 10 minutes | Servings: 4

Ingredients:

1½ teaspoons extra-virgin olive oil

1 cup chopped bell peppers, any color (about 1 medium pepper)

2 garlic cloves, minced (about 1 teaspoon)

6 large eggs

¼ teaspoon kosher or sea salt

2 tablespoons water

½ cup crumbled goat cheese (about 2 ounces)

2 tablespoons loosely packed chopped fresh mint

Directions:

In a large skillet over medium-high heat, heat the oil. Add the peppers and cook for 5 minutes, stirring occasionally. Add the garlic and cook for 1 minute.

While the peppers are cooking, in a medium bowl, whisk together the eggs, salt, and water.

Turn the heat down to medium-low. Pour the egg mixture over the peppers. Let the eggs cook undisturbed for 1 to 2 minutes, until they begin to set on the bottom. Sprinkle with the goat cheese.

Cook the eggs for about 1 to 2 more minutes, stirring slowly, until the eggs are soft-set and custardy. (They will continue to cook off the stove from the residual heat in the pan.)

Top with the fresh mint and serve.

Nutrition:

Calories: 201, Total Fat: 15g, Saturated Fat: 6g, Cholesterol: 294mg, Sodium: 176mg, Total Carbohydrates: 5g Fiber: 2g Protein: 15g

Marinara Eggs With Parsley

Preparation Time: 5 minutes | Cooking Time: 15 minutes | Servings: 6

Ingredients:

1 tablespoon extra-virgin olive oil

1 cup chopped onion (about ½ medium onion)

2 garlic cloves, minced (about 1 teaspoon)

2 (14.5-ounce) cans Italian diced tomatoes, undrained, no salt added

6 large eggs

½ cup chopped fresh flat-leaf (Italian) parsley

Crusty Italian bread and grated Parmesan or Romano cheese, for serving (optional)

Directions:

In a large skillet over medium-high heat, heat the oil. Add the onion and cook for 5 minutes, stirring occasionally. Add the garlic and cook for 1 minute.

Pour the tomatoes with their juices over the onion mixture and cook until bubbling, 2 to 3 minutes. While waiting for the tomato mixture to bubble, crack one egg into a small custard cup or coffee mug.

When the tomato mixture bubbles, lower the heat to medium. Then use a large spoon to make six indentations in the tomato mixture. Gently pour the first cracked egg into one indentation and repeat, cracking the remaining eggs, one at a time, into the custard cup and pouring one into each indentation. Cover the skillet and cook for 6 to 7 minutes, or until the eggs are done to your liking (about 6 minutes for soft-cooked, 7 minutes for harder cooked).

Top with the parsley, and serve with the bread and grated cheese, if desired.

Nutrition:

Calories: 122, Total Fat: 7g, Saturated Fat: 2g, Cholesterol: 186mg, Sodium: 207mg, Total Carbohydrates: 7g Fiber: 1g Protein: 7g

Italian Breakfast Bruschetta

Preparation Time: 10 minutes | Cooking Time: 20 minutes | Servings: 4

Ingredients:

¼ teaspoon kosher or sea salt

6 cups broccoli rabe, stemmed and chopped (about 1 bunch)

1 tablespoon extra-virgin olive oil

2 garlic cloves, minced (about 1 teaspoon)

1 ounce prosciutto, cut or torn into ½-inch pieces

¼ teaspoon crushed red pepper

Nonstick cooking spray

3 large eggs

1 tablespoon 2% milk

¼ teaspoon freshly ground black pepper

4 teaspoons grated Parmesan or Pecorino Romano cheese

1 garlic clove, halved

8 (¾-inch-thick) slices baguette-style whole-grain bread or 4 slices larger Italian-style whole-grain bread

Directions:

Bring a large stockpot of water to a boil. Add the salt and broccoli rabe, and boil for 2 minutes. Drain in a colander. In a large skillet over medium heat, heat the oil. Add the garlic, prosciutto, and crushed red pepper, and cook for 2 minutes, stirring often. Add the broccoli rabe and cook for an additional 3 minutes, stirring a few times. Transfer to a bowl and set aside. Place the skillet back on the stove over low heat and coat with nonstick cooking spray. In a small bowl, whisk together the eggs, milk, and pepper. Pour into the skillet. Stir and cook until the eggs are soft scrambled, 3 to 5 minutes. Add the broccoli rabe mixture back to the skillet along with the cheese. Stir and cook for about 1 minute, until heated through. Remove from the heat.

Toast the bread, then rub the cut sides of the garlic clove halves onto one side of each slice of the toast. (Save the garlic for another recipe.) Spoon the egg mixture onto each piece of toast and serve.

Nutrition:

Calories: 216 Total Fat: 9g, Saturated Fat: 2g Cholesterol: 145mg Sodium: 522mg, Total Carbohydrates: 20g Fiber: 5g Protein: 13g

Julene's Green Juice

Preparation Time: 5 minutes | Cooking Time: 0 minutes | Servings: 1

Ingredients:

3 cups dark leafy greens

1 cucumber

¼ cup fresh Italian parsley leaves

¼ pineapple, cut into wedges

½ green apple

½ orange - ½ lemon

Pinch grated fresh ginger

Directions:

Using a juicer, run the greens, cucumber, parsley, pineapple, apple, orange, lemon, and ginger through it, pour into a large cup, and serve.

Nutrition:

Calories: 108, Protein: 11g Total Carbohydrates: 29g Fiber: 9g Total Fat: 2g

Chapter 12

Lunch Recipes

Italian Lamb Shanks

Preparation Time: 15 minutes | Cooking Time: 60 minutes | Servings: 4

Ingredients:

3 lbs. lamb shanks

4 cloves garlic, minced

3 stalks celery, diced

1 cup beef stock

1 tablespoon balsamic vinegar

1 tablespoon coconut oil

1 tablespoon tomato paste

1 yellow onion, diced

½ teaspoon crushed red pepper flakes

½ teaspoon salt

¼ teaspoon black pepper

1 can (14-ounces) fire-roasted tomatoes

3 carrots, peeled and chopped

Italian parsley, fresh, chopped for garnish

Directions:

Sprinkle lamb shanks with pepper and salt. Set your instant pot to the sauté mode, add the coconut oil and heat.

Add the lamb shanks to hot coconut oil and cook for about 10-minutes or until all sides are brown.

Transfer to a platter when sides are browned.

Add garlic, celery, onion, and carrots to instant pot. Use salt and pepper to season, cook until the onion becomes translucent—stirring often.

Add the fire-roasted tomatoes and tomato paste. Stir to blend.

Return the lamb shanks to the pot. Add the beef stock and balsamic vinegar.

Cancel the sauté mode, and cover pot with lid and secure it.

Set the pot to Manual mode, on high, with a cook time of 45-minutes.

When the cook time is completed, release the pressure naturally for 15-minutes.

Transfer the lamb shanks to a serving plate. Ladle sauce over lamb shanks.

Garnish with fresh, chopped parsley and enjoy warm!

Nutrition:

Calories: 257   Total Fat: 11g   Carbs: 9g   Protein: 28g

Beef Goulash

Preparation Time: 15 minutes | Cooking Time: 15 minutes | Servings: 6

Ingredients:

2 lbs. extra lean ground beef

2 tablespoons of sweet paprika

1 tablespoon garlic, minced

1 large sized onion, cut into strips

1 large sized red bell pepper, stemmed and seeded, cut into strips

2 teaspoons olive oil

2 cans of petite tomatoes, diced

4 cups beef stock

½ teaspoon hot paprika

Directions:

Set to your sauté mode and add 2 tablespoons olive oil.

Add ground beef to the pot and keep cooking and stirring until it breaks.

Once the beef is browned, transfer it to another bowl. Slice the stem of the pepper and deseed them. Cut them into strips.

Cut the onions into short strips.

Add teaspoon olive oil to the pot and add onion and pepper.

Add minced garlic, sweet paprika, and cook for 3-minutes.

Add beef stock and tomatoes.

Add ground beef and close and secure the lid, cook on low pressure for 15-minutes on the SOUP mode.

Use the quick-release when cooking is completed.

Serve hot and enjoy!

Nutrition:

Calories: 283, Total Fat: 13g, Carbs: 14g, Protein: 30g

Instant Pot Korean Beef

Preparation Time: 15 minutes | Cooking Time: 6 hours | Servings: 6

Ingredients:

4lbs. roast, cut into strips

¼ teaspoon salt

¼ teaspoon black pepper

1 cup chicken broth

4 tablespoons soy sauce

¼ teaspoon garlic paste

¼ teaspoon ginger

1 pear, chopped

2 cups orange juice

1 tablespoon honey

Directions:

Trim extra fat off the roast, rinse and fully dry.

Season roast with salt and pepper. Set aside.

Set the instant pot to the sauté mode, add olive oil and heat it.

Add the meat to pot and brown on all sides for about 5-minutes. Remove meat from pot and set aside. In the instant pot pour orange juice, soy sauce, garlic, ginger, pear and honey and stir to blend. Cover up the instant pot with lid and set to Manual mode, on high, for a cook time of 45-minutes. When cook time is completed, release the pressure naturally for 15-minutes. Shred the meat using two forks, then serve with rice and enjoy!

Nutrition:

Calories: 490 Total Fat: 24g Carbs: 26g Protein: 41g

Beef Ragu

Preparation Time: 15 minutes | Cooking Time: 55 minutes | Servings: 6

Ingredients:

18-ounces beef chunks

2 tablespoons parsley, fresh,

Chopped, divided

2 bay leaves

2 sprigs of fresh thyme

7-ounces roasted red peppers

28-ounces crushed tomatoes

5 garlic cloves, smashed

1 teaspoon olive oil

Black pepper as needed

1 teaspoon salt

Directions:

Season the beef with salt and pepper. Set your instant pot to the sauté mode, add the oil and heat it. Cook the garlic in a pot and turn to brown.

It will take about 2-minutes, then remove garlic with slotted spoon.

Put the beef in the instant pot and cook a couple of minutes on each side. Add remaining ingredients to the pot.

Keep half of the parsley for later for garnish.

Cook the beef on manual mode, on high, for a cook time of 45-minutes.

When the cook time is completed, release the pressure naturally for 10-minutes.

Remove the bay leaves and discard them. Shred the beef using two forks.

Garnish beef with remaining parsley and serve hot with some pasta.

Nutrition:

Calories: 298, Total Fat: 11g, Carbs: 14g, Protein: 29g

Sloppy Joe with Beef

Preparation Time: 15 minutes | Cooking Time: 30 minutes | Servings: 6

Ingredients:

2 lbs. ground beef

2 tablespoons yellow mustard

2 tablespoons molasses

2 tablespoons apple cider vinegar

15-ounces tomato sauce

½ teaspoon black pepper

1 teaspoon pepper

1 teaspoon cayenne

2 teaspoons salt

2 teaspoons paprika

2 teaspoons smoked paprika

2 teaspoons cumin

8 garlic cloves, minced

2 onions, diced

2 tablespoons olive oil

Chopped cilantro, for garnishing

Directions:

Set your instant pot to the sauté mode, add oil and heat it.

Sauté, the onions in the oil for 5-minutes, then add the garlic, spices and ground beef.

Cook thoroughly until the beef turns brown. Add all the remaining ingredients, stir.

Close the lid to pot and set on the BEAN/CHILI mode, make sure the steam valve is closed.

After 30-minutes the cook time will be completed, release the pressure naturally for 10-minutes.

Serve hot.

Nutrition:

Calories: 304, Total Fat: 12g, Carbs: 16g, Protein: 28g

Beef & Tomato Soup

Preparation Time: 15 minutes | Cooking Time: 55 minutes | Servings: 6

Ingredients:

1 lb. ground beef

1 tablespoon olive oil

1 medium onion, chopped

Black pepper to taste

15-ounces beef broth

15-ounces diced tomatoes

1 teaspoon oregano, dried

1 teaspoon thyme, dried

1 tablespoon garlic, minced

Directions:

Turn your instant pot to the sauté mode, add the oil and heat it.

Add the beef to pot and cook it until it turns brown.

Add the onion, thyme, oregano, garlic and cook for an additional 3-minutes.

Add the tomatoes and beef broth and close the pot lid. Set to SOUP mode and cook for 30-minutes. When cooking is completed, release the pressure using the quick-release.

Season with salt and pepper.

Serve the soup warm.

Nutrition:

Calories: 302 Total Fat: 15g Carbs: 14g Protein: 30g

Ground Lamb Curry

Preparation Time: 15 minutes | Cooking Time: 55 minutes | Servings: 4

Ingredients:

1 lb. ground lamb

½ teaspoon Kashmiri chili powder

½ teaspoon cumin powder

1 teaspoon salt

1 teaspoon paprika

1 teaspoon meat masala, homemade

1 tablespoon coriander powder

1 onion, diced

1 cup frozen peas, rinsed

2 potatoes, chopped

1 can (13.5-ounce) tomato sauce

3 carrots, chopped

4 tomatoes, chopped

4 garlic cloves, minced

2 tablespoons ghee

1-inch fresh ginger, minced

2 Serrano peppers, minced

¼ teaspoon turmeric powder

½ teaspoon black pepper

Fresh cilantro, chopped for garnish

Directions:

Set your instant pot to the sauté mode, add the ghee and heat it. Add onions and cook them until they start to brown.

Add the garlic, ginger, Serrano pepper and stir-fry for 1-minute. Add the tomatoes. Cook for 5-minutes, then add the spice and stir-fry for 1-minute.

Add the ground lamb and cook until the meat is browned. Add the potatoes, carrots, peas, and tomato sauce. Mix well until combined.

Press the CANCEL button to stop the sauté mode.

Cover and secure the lid to the pot.

Press the CHILI button and cook for 30-minutes.

When the instant pot completes the cooking, release the pressure naturally for 15-minutes. Carefully open the lid and serve dish warm.

Nutrition:

Calories: 267 Total Fat: 8g Carbs: 12g Protein: 27g

Rosemary Lamb

Preparation Time: 15 minutes

Cooking Time: 35 minutes

Servings: 6

Ingredients:

4 lbs. lamb, cubed, boneless

1 cup sliced carrots

2 tablespoons olive oil

3 tablespoons flour

6 rosemary sprigs

4 garlic cloves, minced

Salt and pepper to taste

1 ½ cups veggie stock

Directions:

Set your instant pot to the sauté mode, add the oil and heat.

Season the lamb with salt and pepper. Place lamb inside the pot with minced garlic. Cook until the lamb has browned all over. Add the flour and stir, slowly pour in the stock.

Add the rosemary and carrots, close and secure the pot lid.

Set to Manual mode, on high, with a cook time of 20-minutes.

When the cook time is completed, release the pressure naturally for 10-minutes.

Remove the rosemary stems from the pot.

Serve lamb with plenty of sauce.

Nutrition:

Calories: 272, Total Fat: 11g, Carbs: 9g, Protein: 29g

Thyme Lamb

Preparation Time: 15 minutes | Cooking Time: 55 minutes | Servings: 8

Ingredients:

1 cup fresh thyme

2 lbs. lamb

1 teaspoon oregano

1 tablespoon olive oil

1 tablespoon turmeric

¼ cup chicken stock

4 tablespoons butter

1 teaspoon sugar

¼ cup rice wine

1 teaspoon paprika

1 tablespoon ground black pepper

Directions:

Chop the fresh thyme and combine it with the oregano, ground black pepper, paprika, sugar, rice wine, chicken stock, and turmeric, mix well.

Sprinkle the lamb with the spice mixture and stir carefully.

Transfer the lamb mixture to your instant pot and add olive oil to the pot.

Close the instant pot and secure the lid, set on MEAT mode for 45-minutes.

When the cooking is completed, release the pressure naturally for 10-minutes.

Chill the lamb for a little bit before you slice it.

Serve warm or cold.

Nutrition:

Calories: 282 Total Fat: 12g Carbs: 8g Protein: 28g

Garlic Lamb Shanks with Port

Preparation Time: 15 minutes | Cooking Time: 60 minutes | Servings: 4

Ingredients:

4 lbs. lamb shanks

1 cup port wine

1 cup chicken broth

1 teaspoon rosemary, dried

2 teaspoons balsamic vinegar

2 tablespoons ghee

2 tablespoons tomato paste

20 peeled, whole garlic cloves

Salt and pepper to taste

Directions:

Trim any excess fat from lamb that you do not want, and season it generously with salt and pepper. Heat oil in your instant pot on the sauté mode.

Place the lamb into the pot, and brown it all over.

Pour in the port and stock, stir in the tomato paste and rosemary.

When the tomato paste is dissolved, close and secure the pot lid.

Set to Manual mode, on high, with a cook time of 32-minutes.

When the cook time is completed, release the pressure naturally for 10-minutes.

Remove the lamb from pot and set the pot back onto the sauté mode for about 5-minutes to thicken the sauce.

Add in vinegar and mix well.

Serve with the sauce poured over the lamb.

Nutrition:

Calories: 298 , Total Fat: 13g , Carbs: 11g , Protein: 26g

Sea Bass in a Pan with Peppers

Preparation Time: 15 minutes | Cooking Time: 10 minutes | Servings: 4

Ingredients:

4 sea bass fillet, no skin

2 tablespoons olive oil (for cooking vegetables)

¼ cup olive oil (for cooking fish)

Salt, to taste

1 Red Bell Pepper, cored and chopped

1 Green Bell Pepper, cored and chopped

4 garlic cloves, minced

3 Shallots, chopped

Juice of ½ lemon

½ cup pitted Kalamata olives, chopped

½ tablespoon ground coriander

½ tablespoon garlic powder

1 teaspoon Aleppo pepper (or Sweet Spanish paprika)

1 teaspoon ground cumin

½ teaspoon black pepper

Directions:

Sprinkle fish with salt on both sides and set aside.

Combine the spices in a small bowl to make the spice mixture.

Heat two tablespoons olive oil in a medium-sized skillet over medium-high heat. Add the bell peppers, shallots, and garlic. Season with salt and 1 teaspoon of the spice mixture. Cook, stirring, for 5 minutes.

Reduce the heat, and stir in the halved olives. Leave on low heat while preparing the fish.

Pat fish dry and season with the remaining spice mixture on both sides.

In a large skillet, heat ¼ cup olive oil over medium-high.

Add the fish pieces. Push down on the middle for 30 seconds or so. Cook fish on one side, until nicely browned, about 4-6 minutes.

Carefully turn fish over and cook on other side for 3-4 minutes until nicely browned. Remove fish from heat, immediately drizzle with lemon juice.

Nutrition:

Calories: 312, Protein: 11 g , Fat: 26 g , Carbs: 12 g

Crusty Tuna Patties

Preparation Time: 10 minutes | Cooking Time: 10 minutes | Servings: 4

Ingredients:

2 (5 to 6-ounce) cans tuna, drained cans

½ cup white bread, torn into pieces

2 teaspoons Dijon mustard

1 tablespoon lemon juice

1 teaspoon lemon zest

1 tablespoon water or liquid from tuna

2 tablespoons chopped fresh parsley

2 tablespoons fresh chives, green onions or shallots, chopped

Salt and pepper, to taste

1 egg

A few dashes of Tabasco or Crystal hot sauce

2 tablespoons olive oil

½ teaspoon butter

Directions:

In a medium bowl, mix the tuna, bread, mustard, lemon zest, water, lemon juice, parsley, hot sauce, chives, pepper and salt.

Mix in the egg.

Divide the mixture into four parts. Form each part into a ball and make into a patty.

Place on a wax paper lined tray and chill for one hour.

Heat a little butter and the olive oil in a stick-free or a cast iron skillet on medium high.

Place the patties in the pan carefully, and cook until nicely golden-browned, 3-4 minutes on each side.

Nutrition:

Calories: 130

Protein: 16 g

Fat: 5 g

Carbs: 5 g

Baked Teriyaki Salmon

Preparation Time: 10 minutes | Cooking Time: 20 minutes | Servings: 4

Ingredients:

4 6-ounce salmon fillets

½ white or red onion, chopped

2 bell peppers, chopped

1 cup carrots, sliced

2 cups broccoli florets

Salt and pepper, to taste

2 tablespoons oil

¼ cup soy sauce

1 cup water

2 teaspoons minced garlic

¼ cup packed brown sugar

¼ teaspoon ground ginger

2 tablespoons honey

2 teaspoons sesame seeds

¼ cup cold water

2 tablespoons corn starch

Directions:

Combine soy sauce, water, garlic, ginger, honey, and brown sugar in a medium saucepan and whisk together over medium-high heat. Bring to a boil.

Stir together corn starch and cold water until dissolved, then whisk into boiling sauce and lower heat to medium-low.

Remove from heat, stir in sesame seeds, and let the sauce cool.

Preheat the oven to 420° F.

Grease a baking sheet and place salmon filets in the center.

In a large bowl, mix vegetables with oil, tossing to coat.

Put the vegetables around the salmon. Season everything with pepper and salt.

Drizzle ⅔ of the Teriyaki sauce over the veggies and salmon. Bake for 15-20 minutes, until veggies are easily pierced with a fork and salmon is flaky and tender.

Drizzle with remaining sauce and serve immediately.

Nutrition:

Calories: 201, Protein: 21 g , Fat: 7 g , Carbs: 12 g

Whole Roasted Mackerel

Preparation Time: 5 minutes | Cooking Time: 30 minutes | Servings: 4

Ingredients:

2 whole mackerel, cleaned and gutted

5 sprigs thyme

2 lemons, thinly sliced, cut into half moons

5 sprigs oregano

2 tablespoons olive oil

Salt and pepper, to taste

Directions:

Preheat the oven to 420° F. Line a baking sheet with parchment paper and spray with cooking spray.

Score along one side of the fish. Season scored sections and the cavity with salt and pepper.

Stuff the scored sections with lemon slices, oregano, and thyme.

Stuff the cavities with herbs and remaining lemon slices

Drizzle with olive oil and roast in the oven for 20 minutes, or until golden-brown and the skin is lightly crisp.

Nutrition:

Calories: 126

Protein: 13 g Fat: 8 g   Carbs: 0.2 g

White Fish sautéed with Lemon, Capers and Herbs

Preparation Time: 10 minutes | Cooking Time: 10 minutes | Servings: 4

Ingredients:

2 Tbsp olive oil

2 Tbsp butter

4 large fresh fish fillets

Juice of 2 large lemons

3 Tbsp capers

½ cup chopped fresh parsley, mint, thyme (or any other fresh herbs you like)

Salt and pepper

Directions:

Place a non-stick pan over a medium-high heat and add the olive oil and butter, allow the butter to melt and become slightly frothy

Add the fish to the pan and fry on both sides for about 2 minutes or until golden and almost cooked through

Add the lemon juice and capers, and allow the acid of the lemon juice to deglaze the pan

Add the fresh herbs just before you remove the pan from the heat and serve

Serve with a little extra butter and a wedge of lemon!

Nutrition:

Calories: 282, Protein: 35 g , Fat: 15 g , Carbs: 3 g

Baked Fish with Olives, Tomatoes, and Eggplant

Preparation Time: 10 minutes | Cooking Time: 25 minutes | Servings: 4

Ingredients:

1 eggplant, thinly sliced

4 Tbsp olive oil

Salt and pepper

4 large, fresh white fish fillets

2 cups canned whole tomatoes

20 black olives, (remove the stones if you wish, but not crucial)

Fresh parsley

Directions:

Preheat the oven to 360 degrees Fahrenheit

Lay the eggplant into the bottom of a baking dish, and drizzle each slice with olive oil, salt and pepper and make sure each slice is coated

Pour half of the tomatoes over the eggplant

Lay the fish onto the tomatoes and add the other half of the tomatoes over the top

Scatter the olives over the tomatoes and pop the dish into the oven to bake for about 30 minutes or until the eggplant is soft and the fish is just cooked through

Serve hot, with a scattering of fresh parsley

Nutrition:

Calories: 481

Protein: 60 g

Fat: 19 g

Carbs: 15 g

Grilled White Fish with Fresh Basil Pesto

Preparation Time: 10 minutes | Cooking Time: 20 minutes | Servings: 4

Ingredients:

1 cup fresh basil leaves

4 Tbsp olive oil

¼ cup grated parmesan

¼ cup toasted pine nuts

Juice of ½ lemon

Salt and pepper

4 fresh white fish fillets

Directions:

Place the pesto ingredients into a food processor and blitz until smooth

Place the pesto into a bowl, and add the fish filets, ensuring each one is coated in pestoPlace a griddle pan onto a high heat Place the pesto-coated fish filets onto the hot griddle pan and grill on both sides until slightly charred, and the fish is cooked through but still juicyServe the fish with the leftover pesto on top

Nutrition:

Calories: 488 Protein: 62 g Fat: 25 g Carbs: 1.6 g

White Fish with Chickpeas and Chorizo

Preparation Time: 10 minutes | Cooking Time: 20 minutes | Servings: 4

Ingredients:

2 Tbsp olive oil

4 garlic cloves, finely chopped

1 onion, finely chopped

2 tsp paprika

½ tsp chili powder

5 oz chorizo sausage, sliced

4 large white fresh fish filets

2 cups canned chickpeas (2 cups once drained)

3 large fresh tomatoes, cut into small pieces

Salt and pepper

Fresh coriander/cilantro

Directions:

Place a large sauté pan over a medium-high heat and add the olive oil

Add the garlic and onions to the pan and stir as they soften and become fragrant

Add the paprika, chili, and paprika and stir as the fat in the paprika melts away and the pieces become golden

Shuffle the ingredients in the pan aside to make room for the fish

Add the fish filets to the pan and sprinkle each side with salt and pepper

Cook the fish for about 2 minutes each side until golden

Add the tomatoes and chickpeas to the pan, add more salt and pepper, cover the pan and leave to cook for about 5 minutes

Serve hot, with a generous scattering of coriander/cilantro!

Nutrition:

Calories: 460 Protein: 51 g Fat: 19 g

Fresh Salmon with Lemon Butter and New Potatoes

Preparation Time: 10 minutes | Cooking Time: 20 minutes | Servings: 4

Ingredients:

4 filets fresh salmon

2 lemons, thinly sliced

2 Tbsp butter

Salt and pepper

Fresh parsley, finely chopped

1 ½ lbs new potatoes, halved if they are large, just aim for even-sized pieces

Directions:

Preheat the oven to 400 degrees Fahrenheit and line a baking tray with baking paper

Place the salmon onto the tray and rub each fillet with butter, and sprinkle each with salt and pepper

Lay the lemon slices onto each fillet

Slip the tray into the oven and bake until the salmon is just cooked

Meanwhile, prepare the potatoes: place the potatoes in a large saucepan, sprinkle with a generous dose of salt, and cover with water. Cover, and place over a medium-high heat and allow the water to come to a boil. Once the water is boiling, partially remove the lid and allow the potatoes to simmer until soft

Nutrition:

Calories: 428, Protein: 28 g , Fat: 24 g , Carbs: 29 g

Fresh Fish Puttanesca Salad with Couscous

Preparation Time: 10 minutes | Cooking Time: 15 minutes | Servings: 4

Ingredients:

1 cup couscous (uncooked)

1 Tbsp butter

Salt and pepper

2 Tbsp olive oil

1 ½ lbs fresh white fish, cut into even chunks

1 Tbsp dried chili flakes

Salt and pepper

½ cup roughly chopped fresh basil

4 tomatoes, chopped

25 black olives, pits removed, roughly chopped

4 Tbsp capers

Directions:

In a bowl, add the couscous, butter, salt and pepper. Pour over 1 cup of boiling water, cover, and leave as you prepare the rest of the dish

Add the olive oil to a pan over a medium heat

Add the fish and cook on each side until golden and just cooked through

Add the chili pepper and season with salt and pepper, remove from the heat

Use a fork to fluff the couscous and distribute the butter throughout

Divide the couscous between four serving bowls

In a bow, gently combine the fish, basil, tomatoes, olives, and capers

Divide the fish mixture between the four bowl and spoon over the piles of fluffy couscous

Serve with an extra drizzle of olive oil!

Nutrition:

Calories: 464 Protein: 40 g Fat: 15 g Carbs: 44 g

Tuna Croquettes

Preparation Time: 40 minutes | Cooking Time: 25 minutes | Servings: 8

Ingredients:

6 tablespoons extra-virgin olive oil, plus 1 to 2 cups

5 tablespoons almond flour, plus 1 cup, divided

1¼ cups heavy cream

1 (4-ounce) can olive oil-packed yellowfin tuna

1 tablespoon chopped red onion

2 teaspoons minced capers

½ teaspoon dried dill

¼ teaspoon freshly ground black pepper

2 large eggs

1 cup panko breadcrumbs (or a gluten-free version)

Directions:

In a large skillet, heat 6 tablespoons olive oil over medium-low heat. Add 5 tablespoons almond flour and cook, stirring constantly, until a smooth paste forms and the flour browns slightly, 2 to 3 minutes.

Increase the heat to medium-high and gradually add the heavy cream, whisking constantly until completely smooth and thickened, another 4 to 5 minutes.

Remove from the heat and stir in the tuna, red onion, capers, dill, and pepper.

Transfer the mixture to an 8-inch square baking dish that is well coated with olive oil and allow to cool to room temperature. Cover and refrigerate until chilled, at least 4 hours or up to overnight.

To form the croquettes, set out three bowls. In one, beat together the eggs. In another, add the remaining almond flour. In the third, add the panko. Line a baking sheet with parchment paper.

Using a spoon, place about a tablespoon of cold prepared dough into the flour mixture and roll to coat. Shake off excess and, using your hands, roll into an oval.

Dip the croquette into the beaten egg, then lightly coat in panko. Set on lined baking sheet and repeat with the remaining dough.

In a small saucepan, heat the remaining 1 to 2 cups of olive oil, so that the oil is about 1 inch deep, over medium-high heat. The smaller the pan, the less oil you will need, but you will need more for each batch.

Test if the oil is ready by throwing a pinch of panko into pot. If it sizzles, the oil is ready for frying. If it sinks, it's not quite ready. Once the oil is heated, fry the croquettes 3 or 4 at a time, depending on the size of your pan, removing with a slotted spoon when golden brown. You will need to adjust the temperature of the oil occasionally to prevent burning. If the croquettes get dark brown very quickly, lower the temperature.

Nutrition:

Calories: 245, Protein: 6 g , Fat: 22 g , Carbs: 7 g

Chapter 13

Dinner Recipes

Stuffed Sardines

Preparation Time: 10 minutes | Cooking Time: 10 minutes | Servings: 6

Ingredients:

¼ c. ricotta cheese

¼ c. shredded Pecorino Romano cheese

¼ c. fresh breadcrumbs

¼ c. chopped parsley

3 large eggs

1 lemon

½ tsp. salt

½ tsp. ground pepper

12 Medium sardines

1/3 c. all-purpose flour

2 c. panko breadcrumbs

1 ½ c. olive oil

Directions:

In a medium bowl combine ricotta, Romano, parsley, fresh breadcrumbs, 1 egg, lemon zest, and ¼ teaspoon of salt and pepper. Once thoroughly combined, set aside.

Next, rinse the sardines and pat them dry with a paper towel. Using the remaining salt and pepper season the inside of each sardine, then stuff each with the ricotta mixture.

Place in three separate dishes place the 2 remaining eggs (lightly beaten), flour, and panko. Then using one hand for wet, and the other for a dry dip each sardine in flour, then egg, then panko. Set sardines down on a plate and set aside.

Start to heat the oil in a large cast-iron skillet, over medium-high heat. You want the oil to be shimmering but not smoking. In batches of 2 fry the sardines in the oil until golden brown, approximately 2-4 minutes for each side. Serve immediately with lemon wedges!

Nutrition:

420 calories 19g carbs 26g protein 26g fat

Mini Greek Meatloaves

Preparation Time: 5 minutes | Cooking Time: 25 minutes | Servings: 6

Ingredients:

Nonstick cooking spray

1 tablespoon extra-virgin olive oil

½ cup minced onion (about ¼ onion)

1 garlic clove, minced (about ½ teaspoon)

1 pound ground beef (93% lean)

½ cup whole-wheat bread crumbs

½ cup crumbled feta cheese (about 2 ounces)

1 large egg

½ teaspoon dried oregano, crushed between your fingers

¼ teaspoon freshly ground black pepper

½ cup 2% plain Greek yogurt

⅓ cup chopped and pitted Kalamata olives

2 tablespoons olive brine

Romaine lettuce or pita bread, for serving (optional)

Directions:

Preheat the oven to 400°F. Coat a 12-cup muffin pan with nonstick cooking spray and set aside.

In a small skillet over medium heat, heat the oil. Add the onion and cook for 4 minutes, stirring frequently. Add the garlic and cook for 1 more minute, stirring frequently. Remove from the heat.

In a large mixing bowl, combine the onion and garlic with the ground beef, bread crumbs, feta, egg, oregano, and pepper. Gently mix together with your hands.

Divide into 12 portions and place in the muffin cups. Cook for 18 to 20 minutes, or until the internal temperature of the meat is 160°F on a meat thermometer. While the meatloaves are baking, in a small bowl, whisk together the yogurt, olives, and olive brine. When you're ready to serve, place the meatloaves on a serving platter and spoon the olive-yogurt sauce on top. You can also serve them on a bed of lettuce or with cut-up pieces of pita bread.

Nutrition:

Calories: 244 Total Fat: 13g Saturated Fat: 5g Cholesterol: 87mg Sodium: 355mg Total Carbohydrates: 10g Fiber: 1g Protein: 22g

Yogurt-And-Herb-Marinated Pork Tenderloin

Preparation Time: 6 minutes | Cooking Time: 25 minutes | Servings: 6

Ingredients:

Nonstick cooking spray

2 medium pork tenderloins (10 to 12 ounces each)

½ teaspoon freshly ground black pepper

½ teaspoon kosher or sea salt

¼ cup 2% plain Greek yogurt

1 tablespoon chopped fresh rosemary

Tzatziki yogurt sauce from Chickpea Patties in Pitas (here, step 3) or store-bought tzatziki sauce

1 to 2 tablespoons chopped fresh mint (optional)

Directions:

Preheat the oven to 500°F.

Line a large, rimmed baking sheet with aluminum foil. Place a wire cooling rack on the aluminum foil, and spray the rack with nonstick cooking spray.

Place both pieces of the pork on the wire rack, folding under any skinny ends of the meat to ensure even cooking. Sprinkle both pieces evenly with the pepper and salt.

In a small bowl, mix together the yogurt and rosemary. Using a spoon or your fingers, slather the yogurt mixture over all sides of the pork.

Roast on the wire rack for 10 minutes. Remove the baking sheet from the oven, and turn over both pieces of pork. Roast for 10 to 12 minutes more, or until the internal temperature of the pork measures 145°F on a meat thermometer and the juices run clear. Remove the pork from the rack and place on a clean cutting board. Let rest for 5 minutes, then slice.

While the pork is roasting, make the tzatziki yogurt sauce, adding fresh mint to the sauce, if desired. Serve the sauce with the pork.

Nutrition:

Calories: 183 Total Fat: 10g Saturated Fat: 3g Cholesterol: 73mg Sodium: 372mg Total Carbohydrates: 4g Fiber: 0g Protein: 22g

Rosemary Potatoes

Preparation Time: 10 minutes | Cooking Time: 20 minutes | Servings: 6

Ingredients:

2 lbs baby potatoes

1 fresh rosemary sprig

1 cup vegetable stock

1/4 cup olive oil - 2 garlic cloves

Pepper

Salt

Directions:

Add oil into the inner pot of instant pot and set the pot on sauté mode. Add garlic, potatoes, and rosemary and cook for 10 minutes. Add stock, pepper, and salt and stir well. Seal pot with lid and cook on high for 10 minutes. Once done, release pressure using quick release. Remove lid. Serve and enjoy.

Nutrition:

Calories 163 Fat 8.6 g Carbohydrates 19.4 g Sugar 0.1 g Protein 4 g Cholesterol 0 mg

Delicious Italian Bell Pepper

Preparation Time: 10 minutes | Cooking Time: 13 minutes | Servings: 4

Ingredients:

5 bell peppers, cut into strips

2 tbsp fresh parsley, chopped

1 tbsp garlic, chopped

2 tomatoes, chopped

1 onion, sliced

1 tbsp olive oil

Pepper

Salt

Directions:

Add oil into the inner pot of instant pot and set the pot on sauté mode.

Add onion and sauté for 3 minutes.

Add garlic and bell peppers and cook for 5 minutes.

Add remaining ingredients and stir well.

Seal pot with lid and cook on high for 5 minutes.

Once done, release pressure using quick release. Remove lid.

Stir well and serve.

Nutrition:

Calories 103 Fat 4.1 g, Carbohydrates 17 g Sugar 10.3 g Protein 2.5 g Cholesterol 0 mg

Pesto Zucchini

Preparation Time: 10 minutes | Cooking Time: 8 minutes | Servings: 4

Ingredients:

2 zucchinis, sliced

1 cup vegetable stock

1 tsp Italian seasoning

2 tbsp olive oil

1 cup mozzarella cheese, shredded

1 eggplant, sliced

1 bell pepper, cut into strips

1/4 cup basil pesto

Pepper

Salt

Directions:

Add all ingredients except pesto into the instant pot and stir well.

Seal pot with lid and cook on high for 8 minutes.

Once done, release pressure using quick release. Remove lid.

Stir well. Top with basil pesto and serve.

Nutrition:

Calories 139, Fat 9.1 g, Carbohydrates 12.9 g, Sugar 6.9 g Protein 4.8 g Cholesterol 5 mg

Pesto Cauliflower

Preparation Time: 10 minutes | Cooking Time: 8 minutes | Servings: 2

Ingredients:

2 cups cauliflower florets

1 tbsp olive oil

1 tbsp fresh lemon juice

1/4 cup pine nuts

2 tbsp cream cheese

1/2 cup spinach, chopped

1 avocado, sliced

1/2 tsp red pepper flakes

1/4 tsp dried mint

1/4 tsp dried thyme

1/4 tsp dried rosemary

1 tsp sea salt

Directions:

Add cauliflower into the instant pot. Add water to cover the cauliflower.

Seal pot with lid and cook on high for 5 minutes.

Once done, release pressure using quick release. Remove lid.

Drain cauliflower well and set aside. Clean the instant pot.

Add avocado, spinach, cream cheese, pine nuts, lemon juice, rosemary, thyme, mint, and salt into the blender and blend until smooth.

Add oil into the inner pot of instant pot and set the pot on sauté mode.

Add cauliflower and blended avocado mixture into the pot and stir well and cook for 2 minutes.

Serve and enjoy.

Nutrition:

Calories 445, Fat 42 g, Carbohydrates 17.3 g, Sugar 3.8 g, Protein 7.3 g, Cholesterol 11 mg

Italian Tomato Mushrooms

Preparation Time: 10 minutes | Cooking Time: 13 minutes | Servings: 2

Ingredients:

1 cup tomatoes, chopped

2 cups mushrooms, sliced

1 tbsp olive oil

1/2 cup zucchini, chopped

1/4 cup green onions, chopped

1 cup cream cheese

1/2 tsp mint, chopped

1/2 tsp dried rosemary

1/2 tsp dried oregano

Salt

Directions:

Add tomatoes, rosemary, oregano, mint, and salt into the blender and blend until smooth.

Add oil into the inner pot of instant pot and set the pot on sauté mode.

Add green onion and zucchini and sauté for 5 minutes. Transfer zucchini and onion mixture on a plate.

Add 1 cup water and mushrooms into the pot and stir well.

Seal pot with lid and cook on high for 3 minutes.

Once done, release pressure using quick release. Remove lid.

Add blended tomato mixture, zucchini, and cream cheese and cook on sauté mode for 5 minutes.

Stir well and serve.

Nutrition:

Calories 507 , Fat 48 g , Carbohydrates 11.2 g , Sugar 4.6 g , Protein 12.4 g Cholesterol 128 mg

Chickpea & Potato

Preparation Time: 10 minutes | Cooking Time: 8 minutes | Servings: 2

Ingredients:

1 cup cooked chickpeas

1/2 tsp ground cumin

1 tsp ground coriander

1/4 tsp ginger

2 potatoes, peeled and cubed

1 cup tomatoes, diced

1 onion, chopped

1 tbsp olive oil

1/4 cup vegetable stock

1 tsp turmeric

1/2 tsp salt

Directions:

Add oil into the inner pot of instant pot and set the pot on sauté mode.

Add onion and potatoes and cook for 2-3 minutes.

Add remaining ingredients and stir everything well.

Seal pot with lid and cook on high for 5 minutes.

Once done, allow to release pressure naturally for 10 minutes then release remaining using quick release. Remove lid.

Serve and enjoy.

Nutrition:

Calories 617, Fat 13.7 g , Carbohydrates 104 g, Sugar 18 g, Protein 24.5 g, Cholesterol 0 mg

Zesty Green Beans

Preparation Time: 10 minutes | Cooking Time: 15 minutes | Servings: 4

Ingredients:

1 lb green beans, trimmed

1 cup vegetable stock

1 lemon juice

1 tsp lemon zest, grated

Pepper

Salt

Directions:

Pour the stock into the instant pot.

Add green beans, lemon juice, lemon zest, pepper, and salt into the bowl and toss well.

Transfer green beans into the steamer basket. Place a steamer basket in the pot.

Seal pot with lid and cook on high for 15 minutes.

Once done, allow to release pressure naturally for 5 minutes then release remaining using quick release. Remove lid.

Serve and enjoy.

Nutrition:

Calories 40 Fat 0.3 g, Carbohydrates 8.7 g, Sugar 2.1 g, Protein 2.3 g, Cholesterol 0 mg

Walnut-Rosemary Crusted Salmon

Preparation Time: 10 minutes | Cooking Time: 20 minutes | Servings: 4

Ingredients:

2 teaspoons of Dijon mustard

1 minced clove garlic

¼ teaspoon of lemon zest

½ teaspoon of honey

½ teaspoon of kosher salt

1 teaspoon of chopped fresh rosemary

3 tablespoons of panko breadcrumbs

¼ teaspoon of crushed red pepper

3 tablespoons of finely chopped walnuts

1 pound of frozen or fresh skinless salmon fillet

1 teaspoon of extra-virgin olive oil

Olive oil

Directions:

Preheat the oven to 420°F and use parchment paper to line a rimmed baking sheet.

Combine mustard, lemon zest, garlic, lemon juice, honey, rosemary, crushed red pepper, and salt in a bowl.

Combine walnuts and panko, with oil, in another bowl.

Place the salmon on that baking sheet. Spread that mustard mix on the fish, along with the panko mix. Make sure the fish is adequately coated with the mixtures. Spray olive oil lightly on the salmon.

Bake for about 8-12 minutes (till the salmon can be separated using a fork).

Nutrition:

Carbohydrate – 4 g, Protein – 24 g, Fat – 12 g, Calories: 222 calories

Caprese Stuffed Portobello Mushrooms

Preparation Time: 25 minutes | Cooking Time: 40 minutes | Servings: 2

Ingredients:

3 tablespoons of divided extra-virgin olive oil

1 medium minced clove garlic

½ teaspoon of salt

½ teaspoon of ground pepper

About 14 ounces of Portobello mushrooms, with gills and stems, removed

1 cup of halved cherry tomatoes

A ½ cup of fresh and drained mozzarella pearls patted dry

A ½ cup of thinly sliced fresh basil

2 teaspoons of balsamic vinegar

Directions:

Preheat the oven to 400°F. Combine a ¼ teaspoon of salt, two tablespoons of oil, and a ¼ teaspoon of pepper in a bowl. Use a brush for coating the mushrooms with this mixture.

Place the mushrooms on a baking sheet and bake it for about ten minutes (till the mushrooms get soft).

Stir basil, tomatoes, and mozzarella in a pan. Mix 1 tablespoon of oil, a ¼ teaspoon of salt, and a ¼ teaspoon of pepper in a bowl.

Remove the components of the pan after the mushrooms soften. Fill the mushrooms with the tomato mix.

Bake till the tomatoes wilt and the cheese melts, for about 15 minutes. Drizzle the mushrooms with half teaspoons of vinegar before serving.

Nutrition:

Carbohydrate – 6 g, Protein – 6 g, Fat – 16 g, Calories: 186 calories

Greek Salad Nachos

Preparation Time: 15 minutes | Cooking Time: 15 minutes | Servings: 6

Ingredients:

A ⅓ cup of hummus

2 tablespoons of extra-virgin olive oil

1 tablespoon of lemon juice

¼ teaspoon of ground pepper

3 cups of whole-grain pita chips

1 cup of chopped lettuce

A ½ cup of quartered grape tomatoes

A ¼ cup of crumbled feta cheese

2 tablespoons of chopped olives

2 tablespoons of minced red onion

1 tablespoon of minced fresh oregano

Directions:

Whisk pepper, lemon juice, oil, and hummus in a bowl.

Spread the pita chips on a plate in one layer.

Cover the chips with about ¾ of that hummus mix and top it with tomatoes, red onion, olives, feta, and lettuce. Cover it with the rest of the hummus. Sprinkle oregano on top before serving it.

Nutrition:

Carbohydrate – 13 g, Protein – 4 g, Fat – 10 g, Calories: 159 calories

Greek Chicken with Lemon Vinaigrette and Roasted Spring Vegetables

Preparation Time: 30 minutes | Cooking Time: 50 minutes | Servings: 4

Ingredients:

For the lemon vinaigrette

1 lemon

1 tablespoon olive oil

1 tablespoon crumbled feta cheese

½ teaspoon honey

For the Greek Chicken and roasted veggies

8 ounce of boneless, skinless chicken breast, cut lengthwise in half

A ¼ cup of light mayonnaise

6 cloves of minced garlic

A ½ cup of panko bread crumbs

3 tablespoons of grated Parmesan cheese

½ teaspoon of kosher salt

½ teaspoon of black pepper

1-inch pieces of asparagus, 2 cups

1½ cups of sliced cremini mushrooms

1½ cups of halved cherry tomatoes

1 tablespoon of olive oil

Directions:

To make the vinaigrette, put half teaspoons of zest, one tablespoon of lemon juice, olive oil, cheese, and honey in a bowl.

For the vegetables and chicken, preheat the oven to 470°F. Use a meat mallet for flattening the chicken between two pieces of plastic wrap.

Place the chicken in a bowl and add two garlic cloves and mayonnaise. Mix cheese, bread crumbs, a ¼ teaspoon of pepper, and a ¼ teaspoon of salt together. Dip the chicken in this crumb mix. Spray olive oil over the chicken.

Roast in the oven till the chicken is done and vegetables are tender. Sprinkle dill over it and serve.

Nutrition:

Carbohydrate – 12 g, Protein – 29 g, Fat – 15 g, Calories: 306 calories

Chicken in Tomato-Balsamic Pan Sauce

Ingredients:

2 8-ounce skinless, boneless chicken breasts

½ teaspoon of salt

½ teaspoon of ground pepper

A ¼ cup of white whole-wheat flour

3 tablespoons of extra-virgin olive oil

A ½ cup of halved cherry tomatoes

2 tablespoons of sliced shallot

A ¼ cup of balsamic vinegar

1 cup of low-sodium chicken broth

1 tablespoon of minced garlic

1 tablespoon of toasted and crushed fennel seeds

1 tablespoon of butter

Directions:

Slice the chicken breasts into 4 pieces and beat them with a mallet till it reaches a thickness of a ¼ inch. Use ¼ teaspoons of pepper and salt to coat the chicken.

Heat two tablespoons of oil in a skillet and keep the heat to a medium. Cook the chicken breasts for two minutes on each side. Transfer it to a serving plate and cover it with foil to keep it warm.

Add one tablespoon oil, shallot, and tomatoes in a pan and cook till it softens. Add vinegar and boil the mix till the vinegar gets reduced by half. Put fennel seeds, garlic, salt, and pepper and cook for about four minutes. Remove it from the heat and stir it with butter.

Pour this sauce over chicken and serve.

Nutrition:

Carbohydrate – 9 g, Protein – 25 g, Fat – 17 g, Calories: 294 calories

Chicken Souvlaki Kebabs with Mediterranean Couscous

Preparation Time: 45 minutes | Cooking Time: 2 hours and 20 minutes | Servings: 4

Ingredients:

For the Kebabs-

1 pound of boneless, skinless chicken breast halves in ½-inch strips

1 cup of sliced fennel

⅓ Cup of dry white wine

A ¼ cup of lemon juice

3 tablespoons of canola oil

4 cloves of garlic, minced

2 teaspoons dried and crushed oregano

½ teaspoon salt

¼ teaspoon black pepper

Couscous-

1 teaspoon of olive oil

A ½ cup of Israeli couscous

1 cup of water

A ½ cup of snipped dried tomatoes

A ¾ cup of chopped red sweet pepper

½ cup each of chopped cucumber and red onion

⅓ Cup of plain fat-free Greek yogurt

A ¼ cup of fresh basil leaves, thinly sliced

A ¼ cup of snipped fresh parsley

1 tablespoon of lemon juice

¼ teaspoon of salt

¼ teaspoon of black pepper

Directions:

Place chicken with sliced fennel in a sealable plastic bag and set aside. Combine the lemon juice, white wine, oil, oregano, garlic, pepper, and salt in a bowl for the marinade. Take a ¼ cup of this marinade and set aside.

Pour rest of the marinade over the chicken and refrigerate for 1 ½ hour.

Take wooden skewers and thread chicken on to it in accordion style.

Grill the chicken skewers for six to eight minutes.

Put all the ingredients of couscous in a pan and cook it in olive oil. Serve it alongside the chicken.

Nutrition:

Carbohydrate – 28 g, Protein – 32 g, Fat – 9 g, Calories: 322 calories

Caprese Chicken Hasselback style

Preparation Time: 25 minutes | Cooking Time: 50 minutes | Servings: 4

Ingredients:

2 skinless, boneless chicken breasts - 8 ounces each

½ teaspoon of salt

½ teaspoon of ground pepper

1 medium tomato, sliced

3 ounces of fresh mozzarella, halved and sliced

A ¼ cup of prepared pesto

8 cups of broccoli florets

2 tablespoons of olive oil

Directions:

Preheat the oven to 375°F and coat a rimmed baking sheet with cooking spray.

Make crosswire cuts at half inches in the chicken breasts. Sprinkle pepper and salt on them. Fill the cuts with mozzarella slices and tomato alternatively. Brush both the chicken breasts with pesto and put it on the baking sheet.

Mix broccoli, oil, salt, and pepper in a bowl. Put in the tomatoes if there are any left. Put this mixture on one side of the baking sheet.

Bake till the broccoli is tender, and the chicken is not pink in the center. Cut each of the breasts in half and serve.

Nutrition:

Carbohydrate – 10 g, Protein – 38 g, Fat – 19 g, Calories: 355 calories

Simple Grilled Salmon with Veggies

Preparation Time: 25 minutes | Cooking Time: 25 minutes | Servings: 4

Ingredients:

1 medium zucchini, lengthwise halved

2 orange, red or yellow bell peppers, halved, trimmed, and seeded

1 medium red onion, cut into wedges of 1-inch

1 tablespoon of olive oil

½ teaspoon salt and ground pepper

1¼ pounds salmon fillet, cut into 4 pieces

¼ cup thinly sliced fresh basil

1 lemon, cut into 4 wedges

Directions:

Preheat the grill to medium-high. Brush peppers, zucchini, and onion with oil. Sprinkle a ¼ teaspoon of salt over it. Sprinkle salmon with salt and pepper.

Place the veggies and the salmon on the grill. Cook the veggies for six to eight minutes on each side, till the grill marks appear. Cook the salmon till it flakes when you test it with a fork.

When cooled down, chop the veggies roughly and mix it together in a bowl. You can remove the salmon skin to serve with the veggies. Each serving can be garnished with a tablespoon of basil and a lemon wedge.

Nutrition:

Carbohydrate – 6 g, Protein – 6 g, Fat – 16 g, Calories: 186 calories

Greek Turkey Burgers with Spinach, Feta & Tzatziki

Preparation Time: 30 minutes | Cooking Time: 30 minutes | Servings: 4

Ingredients:

One cup of chopped spinach, frozen and thawed

One pound of lean 93% turkey, ground

Half cup of feta cheese, crumbled

Half tsp. of garlic powder

Half tsp. of oregano, dried

One-fourth tsp. of salt

One-fourth tsp. of pepper, ground

Four hamburger buns, small and whole-wheat

Four tsp. of tzatziki

Twelve slices of cucumber

Eight red onion, thick rings

Directions:

Pre-heat the grill to med-high.

Squeeze moisture from spinach and combine it with turkey, garlic powder, feta, pepper, and salt in a bowl to mix well.

Form 4 four inches of patties and oil the grill rack.

Until cooked, grill patties for four to six minutes for each side until the thermometer reads 165°F.

Assemble burgers on buns and top each with 1 tsp. of tzatziki, two onion rings, and three cucumbers.

Wrap them and refrigerate for eight hours.

Nutrition:

Carbohydrate – 28 g, Protein – 30 g, Fat – 17 g, Calories: 376 calories

Mediterranean Chicken Quinoa Bowl

Preparation Time: 30 minutes | Cooking Time: 30 minutes | Servings: 4

Ingredients:

One pound of skinless and boneless trimmed chicken breasts

One-fourth tsp. of salt

One-fourth tsp. of pepper, ground

1 seven-ounce jar of red pepper, rinsed and roasted

One-fourth cup of almonds, slivered

Four tsps. of olive oil, extra-virgin and divided

Half tsp. of cumin, ground

One-fourth tsp. of red pepper, crushed

Two cups of quinoa, cooked

One-fourth cup of Kalamata olives, pitted and chopped

One-fourth cup of red onion, finely chopped

One cup of cucumber, diced

One-fourth cup of feta cheese, crumbled

Two tsp. of fresh parsley, finely chopped

Directions:

Place a rack in the oven and preheat to lime rimmed baking sheet along with foil

Sprinkle the chicken with pepper and salt to place on the baking sheet. Broil until the thermometer reads 165°F. Then transfer chicken to a cutting board.

Place almonds, oil, pepper, cumin, red pepper, paprika together and puree it.

Combine olives, quinoa, red onion, and the remaining two tablespoons of oil in a bowl.

Before serving, sprinkle the dish with parsley and feta.

Nutrition:

Carbohydrate – 31 g, Protein – 34 g, Fat – 27 g, Calories: 519 calories

Creamy Dill Potatoes

Preparation Time: 10 minutes | Cooking Time: 20 minutes | Servings: 4

Ingredients:

2 lbs potatoes, peeled and cut into chunks

1 tbsp fresh dill, chopped

1 cup vegetable stock

3/4 cup heavy cream

Pepper

Salt

Directions:

Add all ingredients into the inner pot of instant pot and stir well.

Seal pot with lid and cook on high for 20 minutes.

Once done, allow to release pressure naturally for 10 minutes then release remaining using quick release. Remove lid.

Stir and serve.

Nutrition:

Calories 238, Fat 8.6 g, Carbohydrates 37 g, Sugar 2.8 g, Protein 4.5 g, Cholesterol 31 mg

Chapter 14

Snacks Recipes

Mediterranean Flatbread with Toppings

Preparation Time: 10 minutes | Cooking Time: 15 minutes | Servings: 10

Ingredients:

2 medium tomatoes

5 black olives (diced)

8 ounces of crescent rolls

1 clove of garlic (finely chopped)

1 red onion (sliced)

¼ tbs. salt

4 tbs. olive oil

¼ tbs. pepper powder

1 and ½ tbs. Italian seasoning

Parmesan cheese as per requirement

Directions:

Wash and clean the tomatoes properly. Then make very thin and round slices with a sharp knife. You have to ensure that the tomato juices drain out. So, place these on a dry piece of linen cloth.

You will get crescent rolls or flatbread dough in the market. Unroll these and keep these on a big baking tray. Make sure the surface of the baking dish has no grease or water.

Then roll the dough into several portions, which will not be more than 14x10 inches in measurement.

With the help of a rolling pin, shape these into rectangular flatbreads.

Place the tomato slices, diced black olive and onion slices on these flatbreads.

Add the Italian seasoning, olive oil, pepper powder, salt, and chopped garlic together and mix well.

Take the mixture and apply an even coat on all the flatbreads. This mixture will add flavor to the toppings and flatbreads.

Put the baking tray in the microwave oven and set the temperature at 375°.

After 15 minutes, remove the plate from the oven and enjoy your crunchy Mediterranean flatbread with toppings with a glass of red wine.

Nutrition:

Carbohydrate – 9g, Protein - 2g Fat – 6g, Calories: 101

Smoked Salmon and Goat Cheese Bites

Preparation Time: 10 minutes | Cooking Time: 15 minutes | Servings: 12

Ingredients:

8 ounces of goat cheese

1 tbs. of fresh rosemary

2 tbs. of oregano

2 tbs. of basil (fresh)

2 cloves of garlic (chopped)

4 ounces fresh smoked salmon

½ tbs. salt

½ tbs pepper

Directions:

People, living in the Mediterranean regions love to eat fish, especially fatty fish like salmon. This is a classic Mediterranean diet snack that combines the smoky flavors of salmon and the sweet and tanginess of goat cheese.

Put the three herbs on the chopping board and run a knife vigorously through these. Once the herbs have been mixed well, transfer it to a medium sized bowl

The add goat cheese (grated), chopped garlic, pepper and salt in the bowl and mix properly. Keep this mixture for some time to rest.

There are two ways of serving salmon-goat cheese bites. Either you can place a flat piece of smoked salmon on the tray and top it with a dollop of goat cheese and seasoning mix.

The other way is to make small balls with the goat cheese and seasoning mix and wrap a wide stripe of smoked salmon around the ball.

One can also sprinkle some additional Italian seasoning on the final salmon bites to enhance the taste. This step is optional, and omitting it will not mar the original richness of the salmon-cheese bites.

Nutrition:

Carbohydrate – 17.33g, Protein - 54.83g, Fat – 53.33g, Calories: 739

Mediterranean Chickpea Bowl

Preparation Time: 12 minutes | Cooking Time: 13 minutes | Servings: 2

Ingredients:

½ tbs. of cumin seeds

1 large julienned carrot

A ¼ cup of tomatoes (chopped)

1 medium julienned zucchini

A ¼ cup of lemon juice

2 sliced green chilies

¼ cup of olive oil

A ½ cup of chopped parsley leaves

1 minced clove of garlic

¼ tbs. salt

¼ tbs. cayenne pepper powder

A ¼ cup of radish (sliced)

3 tbs. walnuts (chopped)

1/3 feta cheese (crumbled)

1 big can of chickpeas

Proportionate salad greens

Directions:

Another ingredient that you will see on the Mediterranean Diet list is chickpeas. The Mediterranean Chickpea Bowl is a popular snack that can be enjoyed at all times. You can use fresh or canned chickpeas as per preference.

For the salad, you will have to make a special dressing that will make the dish tasty. You need to roast the cumin seeds on a dry pan. Make sure the heat is at medium.

When the seeds begin releasing the aroma, put the seeds in a different mixing bowl.

In this bowl, add the olive oil, garlic, lemon juice, and tomatoes. Also, add the cayenne pepper and salt, and mix well to blend in all the ingredients.

Take a big bowl and add the chickpeas into it. Then put in the sliced and chopped veggies, and parsley leaves.

Adding walnut pieces will add an extra crunch to the Mediterranean chickpea salad.

Put in the seasoning you just prepared and then, mix all the ingredients well.

Nutrition:

Carbohydrate – 30g, Protein - 12g, Fat – 38g, Calories: 492

Hummus Snack Bowl

Preparation Time: 5 minutes | Cooking Time: 5 minutes | Servings: 2

Ingredients:

8 tbs of hummus

½ cup fresh spinach (coarsely chopped)

½ cups of carrots (shredded)

1 big tomato (diced)

¼ tbs. salt

¼ tbs. chili powder

¼ tbs. pepper

6 sweet olives (3 green, 3 black, chopped)

Directions:

The Mediterranean Diet will not be complete without the use of hummus. They don't indulge in fast food, but opt for fresh salad bowls, which are full of nutrition and goodness.

You can either prepare the hummus at home or purchase a jar that does not contain added flavorings and preservatives.

Take a large bowl and put in 6 spoonfuls of hummus into it. In this, put in chopped olives, shredded carrots, spinach leaves, and diced tomatoes.

Coat these vegetables with hummus properly.

After mixing the vegetables and hummus paste for at least five minutes, add in the chili powder. Make sure that it is evenly spread into the whole salad.

Lastly, add pepper powder and salt in the hummus-veggies mixture. You can taste the mixture and check the balance of all the ingredients.

Some also drizzle on some extra virgin olive oil onto the salad. This step is optional and can be omitted.

The Hummus Snack Bowl is a complete snack on its own. If you desire to add some texture to it, some freshly baked flatbreads or bread will complement the salad.

Nutrition:

Carbohydrate – 43g, Protein – 12g, Fat – 10g, Calories: 280

Crock-Pot Paleo Chunky Mix

Preparation Time: 5 minutes | Cooking Time: 1 hour and 30 minutes | Servings: 2

Ingredients:

4 cups of walnuts (raw and roughly broken)

2 cups of cashews (raw and broken in halves)

2 cups of plain coconut flakes

2/3 cups of sugar granules

2 tbs. of olive oil of fresh butter

2 tbs. of extracts of vanilla

12 ounces of dry banana chips

1 and ½ cups of dark chocolate (broken in chips)

Directions:

As the people of the Mediterranean region love to eat nuts, this is one snack that you will find in each household. It is full of good fats and gives you energy and healthy bones. The preparation is rather simple, but the cooking process is lengthy.

To prepare this dish, you will require a medium-sized crock pot.

In this pot, pour in the pieces of walnut, vanilla essence, sugar granules, and olive oil.

After this, you must mix the ingredients well and place the pot on high heat.

Leave the pot at high temperature for around 60 minutes.

After one hour, you need to reduce the heat to low and cook the mixture for another half an hour.

Once the 30 minutes are over, empty the contents of this pot on a dry piece of parchment sheet.

After resting the mix for 15 minutes, you need to put the chocolate chips and banana chips.

Then mix all these ingredients together. The addition of chocolate will add richness to the sweet and nutty snack.

Nutrition:

Carbohydrate – 18.6g, Protein – 4g, Fat – 7g, Calories: 250

Smoked Eggplant Dip

Preparation Time: 20 minutes | Cooking Time: 40 minutes | Servings: 4

Ingredients:

1 and a ½ pound of eggplant

½ tbsp. pepper powder

1 medium coarsely chopped onion

4 tbs. of olive oil

6 peeled cloves of garlic

2 cups of sour cream

¾ tbs. salt

4 tbs. of lemon juice

Fresh parsley (minced)

Liquid smoke (10 drops; optional)

Directions:

Salads, dressing, and dips are predominant in the Mediterranean diet. But not many are aware that eggplant can be used to make a mean dip that will you change the way you view this versatile vegetable.

To start with, you need to peel the outer skin of the eggplants. Using a peeler will come in handy for this task.

As a significant part of the cooking will be done in the oven, it is best to preheat it. Crank up the temperature to 400 degrees.

Make 1-inch thick slices of the eggplant. It will ensure the penetration of flavors and even cooking.

Take an oven baking tray and brush some olive oil onto the pan. Place the eggplant slices on the pan in an orderly fashion.

Sprinkle a thick layer of chopped onions on the eggplant slices. On that, place the cloves of garlic.

Roast the veggies inside the oven for 45 minutes. It is best to bring out the tray once and toss the ingredients.

Once the slices are evenly cooked and cooled, it is time to make a paste in the blender.

When you are happy with the texture of the mixture, add the lemon juice and sour cream into it.

After mixing all the ingredients, put in pepper powder and salt. Adding liquid smoke is optional.

After sprinkling in minced fresh parsley leaves, the dip is ready to be consumed with flatbread or banana chips.

Nutrition:

Carbohydrate – 5g, Protein - 3g, Fat – 5g, Calories: 77

Savory Spinach Feta and Sweet Pepper Muffins

Preparation Time: 10 minutes | Cooking Time: 25 minutes | Servings: 10

Ingredients:

2 and ½ cups of flour

2 tbs. of baking powder

A ¼ cup of sugar

¾ tbs. salt

1 tbs. paprika

A ¾ cup of milk

2 fresh eggs

½ cup olive oil

A ¾ cup of feta (crumbled)

1 and ¼ cups of sliced spinach

1/3 cup of Florina peppers

Directions:

If you are looking for a Mediterranean diet snack that will not only fill your belly but will create an explosion of tastes in your mouth, then this is the ultimate option.

As the muffins will be baked in the oven, you need to preheat it to a temperature of 190 degrees.

Take a deep and large container. In this, put in the sugar, baking powder, salt, and flour. Mix all these dry ingredients properly and make sure there are no lumps.

In a separate container, you need to pour in the milk, eggs and the olive oil. Stir these ingredients so that they form one smooth liquid.

Carefully pour in the liquids in the container that has the dry ingredients. Use your hand to mix everything well, so that a thick and smooth dough is formed.

Then it is time to put in the crumbled feta, pepper and sliced spinach into the dough. Then spend some time with it to ensure that the new ingredients have mixed evenly into the muffin dough.

You can get muffin trays at the market. In such a tray, scoop out portions of the dough and place it into the muffin tray depressions.

Put in this pan inside the oven for 25 minutes. After cooling, the muffins will be ready for consumption.

Nutrition:

Carbohydrate – 15g, Protein – 10g, Fat – 20g, Calories: 240

Italian Oven Roasted Vegetables

Preparation Time: 5 minutes | Cooking Time: 30 minutes | Servings: 4

Ingredients:

2 sliced medium onions

½ tbs. salt

1 tbs. Italian seasoning

2 sliced yellow squash

1/8 tsp pepper powder

3 minced cloves of garlic

2 sweet and large green and red peppers

2 tbs. olive oil

Directions:

Salads form a big part of the Mediterranean diet. The secret to the health and well-being of these people is due to their high vegetable and fruit consumption. If you want to acquire the healthy inner glow, then sacking on these roasted Italian salads will come in handy.

Mixing is an art, and the taste of the salad will depend on how well you mix the ingredients.

Take all the cut, chopped, minced and diced vegetables and put them in a large salad mixing bowl.

After this, you will have to add required amounts of salt, Italian seasoning and pepper powder in the vegetables.

Toss these ingredients for some time to ensure that everything has mixed well.

Then pour in the olive oil into this mixture and again blend well.

Place the marinated vegetables in a roasting oven and put it inside the microwave oven.

The oven must be preheated at 425-degree temperature. The baking will take no longer than 25 minutes.

After pulling out the tray from the oven, you can sprinkle on some extra cheese. This is optional and can be omitted.

Nutrition:

Carbohydrate – 16g, Protein - 3g, Fat – 4g, Calories: 100

Greek Spinach Yogurt Artichoke Dip

Preparation Time: 10 minutes | Cooking Time: 10 minutes | Servings: 2

Ingredients:

1 tbs. olive oil

9-ounces spinach (roughly chopped)

¼ cup Parmesan cheese (grated)

14 ounces Artichoke hearts (chopped)

½ tbsp. pepper powder - ½ tbs. onion powder

½ tbs. garlic powder - 8 ounces sliced chestnuts

2 cups of Greek yogurt (fat-free)

Directions:

Preheat the oven to 350°F. Chop artichoke hearts into bite-sized pieces. Mix all ingredients together and season with a pinch of salt; pour into a small casserole or oven-safe dish (about 1-quart). Sprinkle the top with extra mozzarella cheese. Bake for 20-22 minutes, or until heated through and the cheese on top is melted. Serve warm with pita or tortilla chips.

Nutrition:

Carbohydrate – 20.9 g Protein - 16.3 g Fat – 2.9 g Calories: 170

Sautéed Apricots

Preparation Time: 5 minutes | Cooking Time: *15 Minutes | Servings:* 4

Ingredients:

2 Tablespoons Olive Oil

1 Cup Almonds, Blanched, Skinless & Unsalted

½ Teaspoon Sea Salt, Fine

1/8 Teaspoon Red Pepper Flakes

1/8 Teaspoon Cinnamon, Ground

½ Cup Apricots, Dried & Chopped

Directions:

Place a frying pan over high heat, adding in your almonds, salt and olive oil. Sauté until the almonds turn a light gold, which will take five to ten minutes. Make sure to stir often because they burn easily.

Spoon your almonds into a serving dish, adding in your cinnamon, red pepper flakes, and chopped apricot.

Allow it to cool before serving.

Nutrition:

Calories: 207, Protein: 5 Grams, Fat: 19 Grams, Carbs: 7 Grams

Spiced Kale Chips

Preparation Time: 5 minutes | Cooking Time: *35 Minutes* | *Servings:* 4

Ingredients:

1 Tablespoon Olive Oil

½ Teaspoon Chili Powder

¼ Teaspoon Sea Salt, Fine

3 Cups Kale, Stemmed, Washed & Torn into 2 Inch Pieces

Directions:

Start by heating your oven to 300, and then get out two baking sheets. Line each baking sheet with parchment paper before placing them to the side.

Dry your kale off completely before placing it in a bowl, and add in your olive oil. Make sure the kale is thoroughly coated before seasoning it.

Spread your kale out on your baking sheets in a single layer, baking for twenty-five minutes. Your kale will need roasted halfway through, and it should turn out dry and crispy. Allow them to cool for at least five minutes before serving.

Nutrition:

Calories: 56 Protein, 2 Grams, Fat: 4 Grams, Carbs: 5 Grams

Yogurt Dip

Preparation Time: 5 minutes | Cooking Time: *10 Minutes* | *Servings:* 4

Ingredients:

½ Lemon, Juiced & Zested

1 Cup Greek Yogurt, Plain

1 Tablespoon Chives, Fresh & Chopped Fine

2 Teaspoons Dill, Fresh & Chopped

2 Teaspoons Thyme, Fresh & Chopped

1 Teaspoon Parsley, Fresh & Chopped

½ Teaspoon Garlic, Minced

¼ Teaspoon Sea Salt, Fine

Directions:

Get out a bowl and mix all of your ingredients together until they're well blended. Season with salt before refrigerating. Serve chilled.

Nutrition:

Calories: 59, Protein: 2 Grams, Fat: 4 Grams, Carbs: 5 Grams

Zucchini Fritters

Preparation Time: 5 minutes | Cooking Time: *30 Minutes* | *Servings:* 6

Ingredients:

2 Zucchinis, Peeled & Grated

1 Sweet Onion, Diced Fine

2 Cloves Garlic, Minced

1 Cup Parsley, Fresh & Chopped

½ Teaspoon Sea Salt, Fine

½ Teaspoon Black Pepper

½ Teaspoon Allspice, Ground

2 Tablespoons Olive Oil

4 Eggs, Large

Directions:

Get out a plate and line it with paper towels before setting it to the side.

Get out a large bowl and mix your onion, parsley, garlic, zucchini, pepper, allspice and sea salt together.

Get out a different bowl and beat your eggs before adding them to your zucchini mixture. Make sure it's mixed well.

Get out a large skillet and place it over medium heat. Heat up your olive oil, and then scoop ¼ cup at a time into the skillet to create your fritters. Cook for three minutes or until the bottom sets. Flip and cook for an additional three minutes. Transfer them to your plate so they can drain. Serve with pita bread or on their own.

Nutrition:

Calories: 103, Protein: 5 Grams, Fat: 8 Grams, Carbs: 5 Grams,

Easy Hummus

Preparation Time: 5 minutes | Cooking Time: *5 Minutes* | *Servings:* 6

Ingredients:

3 Cloves Garlic, Crushed

1 Tablespoon Olive Oil

1 Teaspoon Sea Salt, Fine

16 Ounces Canned Garbanzo Beans, Drained

1 ½ Tablespoons Tahini

½ Cup Lemon Juice, Fresh

Directions:

Blend your garbanzo beans, tahini, garlic, olive oil, lemon juice and sea salt together for three to five minutes in a blender. Make sure it's mixed well. It should be fluffy and soft.

Refrigerate for at least an hour before serving with either pita bread or cut vegetables.

Nutrition:

Calories: 187, Protein: 8 Gram, Fat: 7 Grams, Carbs: 25 Grams

Cucumber Bites

Preparation time: 10 minutes | *Cooking time:* 0 minutes | *Servings:* 12

Ingredients:

1 English cucumber, sliced into 32 rounds

10 ounces hummus

16 cherry tomatoes, halved

1 tablespoon parsley, chopped

1 ounce feta cheese, crumbled

Directions:

Spread the hummus on each cucumber round, divide the tomato halves on each, sprinkle the cheese and parsley on to and serve as an appetizer.

Nutrition: calories 162, fat 3.4, fiber 2, carbs 6.4, protein 2.4

Stuffed Avocado

Preparation time: 10 minutes | *Cooking time:* 0 minutes | *Servings:* 2

Ingredients:

1 avocado, halved and pitted

10 ounces canned tuna, drained

2 tablespoons sun-dried tomatoes, chopped

1 and ½ tablespoon basil pesto

2 tablespoons black olives, pitted and chopped

Salt and black pepper to the taste

2 teaspoons pine nuts, toasted and chopped

1 tablespoon basil, chopped

Directions:

In a bowl, combine the tuna with the sun-dried tomatoes and the rest of the ingredients except the avocado and stir.

Stuff the avocado halves with the tuna mix and serve as an appetizer.

Nutrition:

calories 233, fat 9, fiber 3.5, carbs 11.4, protein 5.6

Wrapped Plums

Preparation time: 5 minutes | *Cooking time:* 0 minutes | *Servings:* 8

Ingredients:

2 ounces prosciutto, cut into 16 pieces

4 plums, quartered

1 tablespoon chives, chopped

A pinch of red pepper flakes, crushed

Directions:

Wrap each plum quarter in a prosciutto slice, arrange them all on a platter, sprinkle the chives and pepper flakes all over and serve.

Nutrition: calories 30, fat 1, fiber 0, carbs 4, protein 2

Cucumber Sandwich Bites

Preparation time: 5 minutes | *Cooking time:* 0 minutes | *Servings:* 12

Ingredients:

1 cucumber, sliced

8 slices whole wheat bread

2 tablespoons cream cheese, soft

1 tablespoon chives, chopped

¼ cup avocado, peeled, pitted and mashed

1 teaspoon mustard

Salt and black pepper to the taste

Directions:

Spread the mashed avocado on each bread slice, also spread the rest of the ingredients except the cucumber slices.

Divide the cucumber slices on the bread slices, cut each slice in thirds, arrange on a platter and serve as an appetizer.

Nutrition: calories 187, fat 12.4, fiber 2.1, carbs 4.5, protein 8.2

Cucumber Rolls

Preparation time: 5 minutes | *Cooking time:* 0 minutes | *Servings:* 6

Ingredients:

1 big cucumber, sliced lengthwise

1 tablespoon parsley, chopped

8 ounces canned tuna, drained and mashed

Salt and black pepper to the taste

1 teaspoon lime juice

Directions:

Arrange cucumber slices on a working surface, divide the rest of the ingredients, and roll.

Arrange all the rolls on a platter and serve as an appetizer.

Nutrition:

calories 200, fat 6, fiber 3.4, carbs 7.6, protein 3.5

Olives and Cheese Stuffed Tomatoes

Preparation time: 10 minutes | *Cooking time:* 0 minutes | *Servings:* 24

Ingredients:

24 cherry tomatoes, top cut off and insides scooped out

2 tablespoons olive oil

¼ teaspoon red pepper flakes

½ cup feta cheese, crumbled

2 tablespoons black olive paste

¼ cup mint, torn

Directions:

In a bowl, mix the olives paste with the rest of the ingredients except the cherry tomatoes and whisk well.

Stuff the cherry tomatoes with this mix, arrange them all on a platter and serve as an appetizer.

Nutrition:

calories 136, fat 8.6, fiber 4.8, carbs 5.6, protein 5.1

Tomato Salsa

Preparation time: 5 minutes | *Cooking time:* 0 minutes | *Servings:* 6

Ingredients:

1 garlic clove, minced

4 tablespoons olive oil

5 tomatoes, cubed

1 tablespoon balsamic vinegar

¼ cup basil, chopped

1 tablespoon parsley, chopped

1 tablespoon chives, chopped

Salt and black pepper to the taste

Pita chips for serving

Directions:

In a bowl, mix the tomatoes with the garlic and the rest of the ingredients except the pita chips, stir, divide into small cups and serve with the pita chips on the side.

Nutrition:

calories 160, fat 13.7, fiber 5.5, carbs 10.1, protein 2.2

Chapter 15

Dessert Recipes

Blueberries Stew

Preparation Time: 10 minutes | Cooking Time: 10 minutes | Servings: 4

Ingredients:

2 cups blueberries

3 tablespoons stevia

1 and ½ cups pure apple juice

1 teaspoon vanilla extract

Directions:

In a pan, combine the blueberries with stevia and the other ingredients, bring to a simmer and cook over medium-low heat for 10 minutes.

Divide into cups and serve cold.

Nutrition:

Calories 192, Fat 5.4, Fiber 3.4, Carbs 9.4 Protein 4.5

Mandarin Cream

Preparation Time: 20 minutes | Cooking Time: 0 minutes | Servings: 8

Ingredients:

2 mandarins, peeled and cut into segments

Juice of 2 mandarins

2 tablespoons stevia

4 eggs, whisked

¾ cup stevia

¾ cup almonds, ground

Directions:

In a blender, combine the mandarins with the mandarins juice and the other ingredients, whisk well, divide into cups and keep in the fridge for 20 minutes before serving.

Nutrition:

Calories 106, Fat 3.4, Fiber 0, Carbs 2.4 Protein 4

Creamy Mint Strawberry Mix

Preparation Time: 10 minutes | Cooking Time: 30 minutes | Servings: 6

Ingredients:

Cooking spray

¼ cup stevia

1 and ½ cup almond flour

1 teaspoon baking powder

1 cup almond milk

1 egg, whisked

2 cups strawberries, sliced

1 tablespoon mint, chopped   - 1 teaspoon lime zest, grated

½ cup whipping cream

Directions: In a bowl, combine the almond with the strawberries, mint and the other ingredients except the cooking spray and whisk well. Grease 6 ramekins with the cooking spray, pour the strawberry mix inside, introduce in the oven and bake at 350 degrees F for 30 minutes. Cool down and serve.

Nutrition: Calories 200 Fat 6.3 Fiber 2 Carbs 6.5 Protein 8

Vanilla Cake

Preparation Time: 10 minutes | Cooking Time: 25 minutes | Servings: 10

Ingredients:

3 cups almond flour

3 teaspoons baking powder

1 cup olive oil

1 and ½ cup almond milk

1 and 2/3 cup stevia

2 cups water

1 tablespoon lime juice

2 teaspoons vanilla extract

Cooking spray

Directions:

In a bowl, mix the almond flour with the baking powder, the oil and the rest of the ingredients except the cooking spray and whisk well. Pour the mix into a cake pan greased with the cooking spray, introduce in the oven and bake at 370 degrees F for 25 minutes. Leave the cake to cool down, cut and serve!

Nutrition:

Calories 200 Fat 7.6 Fiber 2.5 Carbs 5.5 Protein 4.5

Pumpkin Cream

Preparation Time: 5 minutes | Cooking Time: 5 minutes | Servings: 2

Ingredients:

2 cups canned pumpkin flesh

2 tablespoons stevia

1 teaspoon vanilla extract

2 tablespoons water

A pinch of pumpkin spice

Directions:

In a pan, combine the pumpkin flesh with the other ingredients, simmer for 5 minutes, divide into cups and serve cold.

Nutrition:

Calories 192, Fat 3.4, Fiber 4.5, Carbs 7.6, Protein 3.5

Chia and Berries Smoothie Bowl

Preparation Time: 5 minutes | Cooking Time: 0 minutes | Servings: 2

Ingredients:

1 and ½ cup almond milk

1 cup blackberries

¼ cup strawberries, chopped

1 and ½ tablespoons chia seeds

1 teaspoon cinnamon powder

Directions:

In a blender, combine the blackberries with the strawberries and the rest of the ingredients, pulse well, divide into small bowls and serve cold.

Nutrition:

Calories 182, Fat 3.4, Fiber 3.4, Carbs 8.4, Protein 3

Minty Coconut Cream

Preparation Time: 4 minutes | Cooking Time: 0 minutes | Servings: 2

Ingredients:

1 banana, peeled

2 cups coconut flesh, shredded

3 tablespoons mint, chopped

1 and ½ cups coconut water

2 tablespoons stevia

½ avocado, pitted and peeled

Directions:

In a blender, combine the coconut with the banana and the rest of the ingredients, pulse well, divide into cups and serve cold.

Nutrition:

Calories 193

Fat 5.4

Fiber 3.4

Carbs 7.6 Protein 3

Watermelon Cream

Preparation Time: 15 minutes | Cooking Time: 0 minutes | Servings: 2

Ingredients:

1 pound watermelon, peeled and chopped

1 teaspoon vanilla extract

1 cup heavy cream

1 teaspoon lime juice

2 tablespoons stevia

Directions:

In a blender, combine the watermelon with the cream and the rest of the ingredients, pulse well, divide into cups and keep in the fridge for 15 minutes before serving.

Nutrition:

Calories 122, Fat 5.7, Fiber 3.2, Carbs 5.3, Protein 0.4

Grapes Stew

Preparation Time: 10 minutes | Cooking Time: 10 minutes | Servings: 4

Ingredients:

2/3 cup stevia

1 tablespoon olive oil

1/3 cup coconut water

1 teaspoon vanilla extract

1 teaspoon lemon zest, grated

2 cup red grapes, halved

Directions:

Heat up a pan with the water over medium heat, add the oil, stevia and the rest of the ingredients, toss, simmer for 10 minutes, divide into cups and serve.

Nutrition:

Calories 122, Fat 3.7, Fiber 1.2, Carbs 2.3 Protein 0.4

Cocoa Sweet Cherry Cream

Preparation Time: 2 hours | Cooking Time: 0 minutes | Servings: 4

Ingredients:

½ cup cocoa powder

¾ cup red cherry jam

¼ cup stevia

2 cups water

1 pound cherries, pitted and halved

Directions:

In a blender, mix the cherries with the water and the rest of the ingredients, pulse well, divide into cups and keep in the fridge for 2 hours before serving.

Nutrition:

Calories 162, Fat 3.4, Fiber 2.4, Carbs 5

Loukoumade (Fried Honey Balls)

Preparation Time: 20 minutes | Cooking Time: 45 minutes | Servings: 10

Ingredients:

2 cups of sugar

1 cup of water

1 cup honey

1 ½ cups tepid water

1 tbsp. brown sugar

¼ cup of vegetable oil

1 tbsp. active dry yeast

1 ½ cups all-purpose flour, 1 cup cornstarch, ½ tsp salt

Vegetable oil for frying

1 ½ cups chopped walnuts

¼ cup ground cinnamon

Directions:

Boil the sugar and water on medium heat. Add honey after 10 minutes. cool and set aside.

Mix the tepid water, oil, brown sugar,' and yeast in a large bowl. Allow it to sit for 10 minutes. In another bowl, mix the flour, salt, and cornstarch. With your hands mix the yeast and the flour to make a wet dough. Cover and set aside for 2 hours.

Fry in oil at 350°F. Use your palm to measure the sizes of the dough as they are dropped in the frying pan. Fry each batch for about 3-4 minutes.

Immediately the loukoumades are done frying, drop them in the prepared syrup.

Serve with cinnamon and walnuts.

Nutrition:

Calories: 355kcal, Carbs: 64g, Fat: 7g, Protein: 6g

Crème Caramel

Preparation Time: 1 hour | Cooking Time: 1 hour | Servings: 12

Ingredients:

5 cups of whole milk

2 tsp vanilla extract

8 large egg yolks

4 large-sized eggs

2 cups sugar, divided

¼ cup 0f water

Directions:

Preheat the oven to 350°F

Heat the milk on medium heat until it is scalded.

Mix 1 cup of sugar and eggs in a bowl and add it to the eggs.

With a nonstick pan on high heat, boil the water and remaining sugar. Do not stir, instead whirl the pan. When the sugar forms caramel, divide it into ramekins.

Divide the egg mixture into the ramekins and place in a baking pan. Add water to the pan until it is half full. Bake for 30 minutes.

Remove the ramekins from the baking pan, cool, then refrigerate for at least 8 hours.

Serve.

Nutrition:

Calories: 110kcal, Carbs: 21g, Fat: 1g, Protein: 2g

Galaktoboureko

Preparation Time: 30 minutes | Cooking Time: 90 minutes | Servings: 12

Ingredients:

4 cups sugar, divided

1 tbsp. fresh lemon juice

1 cup of water

1 Tbsp. plus 1 ½ tsp grated lemon zest, divided into 10 cups

Room temperature whole milk

1 cup plus 2 tbsps. unsalted butter, melted and divided into 2

Tbsps. vanilla extract

7 large-sized eggs

1 cup of fine semolina

1 package phyllo, thawed and at room temperature

Directions:

Preheat oven to 350°F

Mix 2 cups of sugar, lemon juice, 1 ½ tsp of lemon zest, and water. Boil over medium heat. Set aside.

Mix the milk, 2 Tbsps. of butter, and vanilla in a pot and put on medium heat. Remove from heat when milk is scalded

Mix the eggs and semolina in a bowl, then add the mixture to the scalded milk. Put the egg-milk mixture on medium heat. Stir until it forms a custard-like material.

Brush butter on each sheet of phyllo and arrange all over the baking pan until everywhere is covered. Spread the custard on the bottom pile phyllo

Arrange the buttered phyllo all over the top of the custard until every inch is covered.

Bake for about 40 minutes. cover the top of the pie with all the prepared syrup. Serve.

Nutrition:

Calories: 393kcal, Carbs: 55g, Fat: 15g, Protein: 8g

Kourabiedes Almond Cookies

Preparation Time: 20 minutes | Cooking Time: 50 minutes | Servings: 20

Ingredients:

1 ½ cups unsalted butter, clarified, at room temperature 2 cups

Confectioners' sugar, divided

1 large egg yolk

2 tbsps. brandy

1 1/2 tsp baking powder

1 tsp vanilla extract

5/ cups all-purpose flour, sifted

1 cup roasted almonds, chopped

Directions:

Preheat the oven to 350°F

Thoroughly mix butter and ½ cup of sugar in a bowl. Add in the egg after a while. Create a brandy mixture by mixing the brandy and baking powder. Add the mixture to the egg, add vanilla, then keep beating until the ingredients are properly blended

Add flour and almonds to make a dough.

Roll the dough to form crescent shapes. You should be able to get about 40 pieces. Place the pieces on a baking sheet, then bake in the oven for 25 minutes.

Allow the cookies to cool, then coat them with the remaining confectioner's sugar.

Serve.

Nutrition:

Calories: 102kcal, Carbs: 10g, Fat: 7g, Protein: 2g

Ekmek Kataifi

Preparation Time: 30 minutes | Cooking Time: 45 minutes | Servings: 10

Ingredients:

1 cup of sugar

1 cup of water

2 (2-inch) strips lemon peel, pith removed

1 tbsp. fresh lemon juice

½ cup plus 1 tbsp. unsalted butter, melted

½lbs. frozen kataifi pastry, thawed, at room temperature

2 ½ cups whole milk

½ tsp. ground mastiha

2 large eggs

¼ cup fine semolina

1 tsp. of cornstarch

¼ cup of sugar

½ cup sweetened coconut flakes

1 cup whipping cream

1 tsp. vanilla extract

1 tsp. powdered milk

3 tbsps. of confectioners' sugar

½ cup chopped unsalted pistachios

Directions:

Set the oven to 350°F. Grease the baking pan with 1. Tbsp of butter.

Put a pot on medium heat, then add water, sugar, lemon juice, lemon peel. Leave to boil for about 10 minutes. Reserve.

Untangle the kataifi, coat with the leftover butter, then place in the baking pan.

Mix the milk and mastiha, then place it on medium heat. Remove from heat when the milk is scalded, then cool the mixture.

Mix the eggs, cornstarch, semolina, and sugar in a bowl, stir thoroughly, then whisk the cooled milk mixture into the bowl.

Transfer the egg and milk mixture to a pot and place on heat. Wait for it to thicken like custard, then add the coconut flakes and cover it with a plastic wrap. Cool.

Spread the cooled custard-like material over the kataifi. Place in the refrigerator for at least 8 hours.

Strategically remove the kataifi from the pan with a knife. Remove it in such a way that the mold faces up.

Whip a cup of cream, add 1 tsp. vanilla, 1tsp. powdered milk, and 3 tbsps. Of sugar. Spread the mixture all over the custard, wait for it to harden, then flip and add the leftover cream mixture to the kataifi side.

Nutrition:

Calories: 649kcal, Carbs: 37g, Fat: 52g, Protein: 11g

Revani Syrup Cake

Preparation Time: 30 minutes | Cooking Time: 3 hours | Servings: 24

Ingredients:

1 tbsp. unsalted butter

2 tbsps. all-purpose flour

1 cup ground rusk or bread crumbs

1 cup fine semolina flour

¾ cup ground toasted almonds

3 tsp baking powder

16 large eggs

2 tbsps. vanilla extract

3 cups of sugar, divided

3 cups of water

5 (2-inch) strips lemon peel, pith removed

3 tbsps. fresh lemon juice

1 oz of brandy

Directions:

Preheat the oven to 350°F. Grease the baking pan with 1 Tbsp. of butter and flour.

Mix the rusk, almonds, semolina, baking powder in a bowl.

In another bowl, mix the eggs, 1 cup of sugar, vanilla, and whisk with an electric mixer for about 5 minutes. Add the semolina mixture to the eggs and stir.

Pour the stirred batter into the greased baking pan and place in the preheated oven.

With the remaining sugar, lemon peels, and water make the syrup by boiling the mixture on medium heat. Add the lemon juice after 6 minutes, then cook for 3 minutes. Remove the lemon peels and set the syrup aside.

After the cake is done in the oven, spread the syrup over the cake.

Cut the cake as you please and serve.

Nutrition:

Calories: 348kcal, Carbs: 55g, Fat: 9g, Protein: 5g

Almonds and Oats Pudding

Preparation Time: 10 minutes | Cooking Time: 15 minutes | Servings: 4

Ingredients:

1 tablespoon lemon juice

Zest of 1 lime

1 and ½ cups almond milk

1 teaspoon almond extract

½ cup oats

2 tablespoons stevia

½ cup silver almonds, chopped

Directions:

In a pan, combine the almond milk with the lime zest and the other ingredients, whisk, bring to a simmer and cook over medium heat for 15 minutes.

Divide the mix into bowls and serve cold.

Nutrition:

Calories 174, Fat 12.1, Fiber 3.2, Carbs 3.9, Protein 4.8

Chocolate Cups

Preparation Time: 2 hours | Cooking Time: 0 minutes | Servings: 6

Ingredients:

½ cup avocado oil

1 cup, chocolate, melted

1 teaspoon matcha powder

3 tablespoons stevia

Directions:

In a bowl, mix the chocolate with the oil and the rest of the ingredients, whisk really well, divide into cups and keep in the freezer for 2 hours before serving.

Nutrition:

Calories 174, Fat 9.1, Fiber 2.2, Carbs 3.9, Protein 2.8

Mango Bowls

Preparation Time: 30 minutes | Cooking Time: 0 minutes | Servings: 4

Ingredients:

3 cups mango, cut into medium chunks

½ cup coconut water

¼ cup stevia

1 teaspoon vanilla extract

Directions:

In a blender, combine the mango with the rest of the ingredients, pulse well, divide into bowls and serve cold.

Nutrition:

Calories 122, Fat 4, Fiber 5.3, Carbs 6.6, Protein 4.5

Cocoa and Pears Cream

Preparation Time: 10 minutes | Cooking Time: 0 minutes | Servings: 4

Ingredients:

2 cups heavy creamy

1/3 cup stevia

¾ cup cocoa powder

6 ounces dark chocolate, chopped

Zest of 1 lemon

2 pears, chopped

Directions:

In a blender, combine the cream with the stevia and the rest of the ingredients, pulse well, divide into cups and serve cold.

Nutrition:

Calories 172, Fat 5.6, Fiber 3.5, Carbs 7.6 Protein 4

Pineapple Pudding

Preparation Time: 10 minutes | Cooking Time: 40minutes | Servings: 4

Ingredients:

3 cups almond flour

¼ cup olive oil

1 teaspoon vanilla extract

2 and ¼ cups stevia

3 eggs, whisked

1 and ¼ cup natural apple sauce

2 teaspoons baking powder

1 and ¼ cups almond milk - 2 cups pineapple, chopped

Cooking spray

Directions:

In a bowl, combine the almond flour with the oil and the rest of the ingredients except the cooking spray and stir well.

Grease a cake pan with the cooking spray, pour the pudding mix inside, introduce in the oven and bake at 370 degrees F for 40 minutes. Serve the pudding cold.

Nutrition:

Calories 223, Fat 8.1, Fiber 3.4, Carbs 7.6

Conclusion

As you can now see, the Mediterranean diet is not a restrictive one and it's so easy to follow.

You can eat so many wonderful and delicious dishes and you can use so many different and versatile ingredients to make them.

The Mediterranean diet will change the way you look in a matter of days. It will improve your overall health, your metabolism and it will help you lose the extra weight.

This recipes collection you've just discovered is full of delicious meals you can try at home. All these recipes taste divine and you will definitely be impressed with the textures and flavors.

So, what are you waiting for? Get your hands on a copy of this great Mediterranean diet recipes collection and make some incredible culinary feasts for all your loved ones.

Enjoy all these intense flavors and have fun discovering the Mediterranean diet!

Dash Diet Cookbook

21-Day Mediterranean Dash Diet Meal Plan to Improve your Health and Lose Weight with Easy and Quick Recipes. With More Than 125 Delectable Recipes!

Marla Smith

Introduction

The DASH diet is an ideal way to quickly bring down your blood pressure through correcting bad eating habits. Even though the approach shows a much healthier eating plan it's still important not to overeat. If you're planning on following the DASH for weight loss then you can be a little more flexible with your foods but you'll want to be stricter with your calories.

Within 2 Weeks you should see an improvement in your blood pressure numbers and potentially some weight loss. Make sure you're keeping hydrated to flush out excess sodium.

Potassium, Magnesium, Calcium, and Whole grains are all important in the DASH approach so try and find foods that are rich in these nutrients. Stay away from added sugar and salt as much as possible.

The reason the DASH approach is so successful in such a short time is that it's making sure your body has the nutrients it needs and avoiding the products that aggravate the problem. Don't forget to plan ahead for times when you might consider snacking.

Remember, the DASH approach isn't about denying you any of the foods you want, simply making healthier choices or versions of them. If you happen to have a day where you haven't been strict don't worry about it. A cheat day does everyone good, just try not to make it too often.

Exercise and a healthy lifestyle are also part of the DASH approach, if you're tweaking your diet why not tweak other things too that can really make a big impact on your numbers.

Even if you don't stick to the meal plans hopefully you've gotten enough information to learn more about the DASH diet and what you should be doing to form your own. With all this information you're sure to see a quick improvement in your numbers.

What is the DASH Diet?

I'm sure you've been through diets in your life. If not you, you must have known people who begin a diet enthusiastically, then hit a plateau and give it all up in frustration and resume their unhealthy eating habits. Wondering what the DASH diet is all about? It's a one of a kind diet, specifically designed to reduce blood pressure levels in people. Hypertension, or high blood pressure, is one of the greatest silent killers of this century.

The DASH diet is rich in fruits, vegetables, whole grains, and low-fat dairy products. Its emphasis isn't on deprivation, but on adaptation. The DASH diet aims to change the way people look at food, to educate them about their bodies, and to teach them to make healthy, sustainable choices.

The DASH diet was created to change lives by changing lifestyles. Unlike more restrictive diets, the DASH diet was designed to be approachable, and to be readily incorporated into people's lives. For the most part, you do not need to shop at special grocery stores or go through agonizing transition periods; you just need to start adjusting your food patterns, one step at a time.

The basics of the DASH diet are simple: Eat more fruits, vegetables, whole grains, and lean protein, and eat less saturated fat, salt, and sweets. It's a common-sense approach to health that really works.

Why The Dash Diet Works

The DASH diet works because it's a lifestyle that can be sustained easily, not a traditional diet. The word "diet" conjures thoughts of temporary deprivation, but the DASH diet is the opposite. It aims at educating individuals on how they can undertake clean or proper eating, on a daily basis, so that they build healthy bodies. Rather than impose strict controls on food content, such as the total number of fats, DASH diet follows important rules of choosing clean foods. When individuals understand the implications of their daily dietary decision making, they're much more likely to choose wisely. Therefore, it is easy to adopt the DASH diet.

The ultimate goal of the DASH diet is to reduce the intake of harmful foods and to choose healthy substitutes instead. When you understand the damage that bad food does to your body, it makes you far less interested in eating it. And once you wean yourself from excess fat, cholesterol, sodium, and sugar, you will be amazed by how much better you feel! Bad food takes its toll in so many ways, not just silently with hypertension and heart disease, but also outwardly in your appearance, energy level, and enthusiasm for life. If you are feeling sluggish, consider what you last ate. Was it good for you? Or bad? Unless you are fueling your body with good food, it will fail you. The DASH diet isn't a strict dietary regimen, but rather a new way of seeing, appreciating, and consuming food.

Grains, vegetables, fruits, low-fat dairy products, seeds, nuts, and lean meat all form the base of the DASH diet. So, there are no strict restrictions, only amazing benefits. Besides giving you a way of turning to healthy eating habits, the DASH diet is primarily known for showing great results in lowering high blood pressure. This diet is rich in several minerals like calcium, zinc, iron, manganese, and potassium, and these nutrients primarily help to regulate the blood pressure. Also, the diet is low in saturated fat and cholesterol but provides a significant amount of protein, which can also help people suffering from high blood pressure.

Knowing what kind of foods make the foundation of this diet makes it clear that it can also be used to lose weight and excess fat. Following this kind of diet means losing about 500 calories a day. Combine that with exercise, and you will get slim fast. What supports this is also the fact that the DASH diet, rich in protein and fiber, keeps you satiated for longer periods and thus prevents overeating and gaining weight.

The DASH diet is one of the few diets that can help you meet your daily requirement for potassium, which, besides countering the effect of salt to raise blood pressure, also helps in preventing osteoporosis. This diet also provides sufficient amounts of vitamin B 12, calcium, and fiber, which are required for proper cell metabolism, building and maintaining strong bones, keeping blood sugar levels stable, and preventing obesity.

DASH Diet Health Plan

Dash diet for high blood pressure/hypertension

Your daily sodium intake from food should be between 1500 and 2300 milligrams per day. The latter is the highest level of sodium that is acceptable according to the National High Blood Pressure Education Program. This is also the amount that is recommended by the US Dietary Guidelines for Americans. 1500 Milligrams is the ideal amount of sodium per day according to the Institute of Medicine. This is the level that you should eventually strive for.

Blood pressure will gradually reduce as you reduce the amount of sodium you consume. DASH menus usually contain 2300 milligrams of sodium to help lower blood pressure gradually. On average, most men consume close to 4200 milligrams of sodium and women consume 3300 milligrams of sodium per day – which is significantly higher than the suggested levels.

The DASH diet consists of food that is low in sodium suitable for patients suffering from blood pressure. With DASH diet, you will experience multiple benefits that you can help you stabilize your blood pressure levels. When you follow a combination of a balanced eating plan and also work towards reducing the sodium content in food, you will be able to prevent the development of high blood pressure.

Dash diet for weight loss

Dash Diet indeed helps to trim your weight by various indirect means.

While the DASH diet does not focus on reducing calories, it fills up your diet with very nutrient dense foods as opposed to ones that are rich in calories, this helps to shed off a few pounds!

This diet is a great way to lose weight because it incorporates fresh, whole foods and reduces packaged, processed foods that are filled with empty calories. Not only will you lose weight, you'll also have a better chance of keeping it off. DASH goes beyond the calorie counting and helps you establish sound eating habits that improve your chances for maintaining healthy weight.

Being on a diet full of veggies and fruits, you will consume lots of fiber, which is also believed to help in weight loss.

Apart from that, the diet also controls your appetite since cleaner and nutrition dense foods will keep you satisfied throughout the whole day. Lowering the food intake will further contribute to weight loss.

Steps towards Transitioning to the DASH Diet

Changing your eating habits needs to be done gradually. Here are a few suggestions to help you make an easy transition to the DASH diet:

Keep a journal and track your eating habits. What do you eat for breakfast, lunch, and dinner? How often do you eat in between meals, and what are you snacking on? From your journal, you can figure out where you need to make changes. For example, add a cup or two of vegetables and fruits to help reduce too many servings of meat. Limit your sodium and sugar by reading the nutrition facts labels on food packages.

When shopping, choose "low-fat," "non-fat," "no sugar added," "no cholesterol," and other healthier versions of products. For grain servings, choose whole grains, such as whole wheat bread and whole grain cereals.

If you love butter or margarine, decrease the amount you use by half and switch to no-cholesterol and low-sodium versions. You can use spices as a substitute for salt. Experiment with different herbs if you're not sure how they taste. Some examples of spices you can try are rosemary, basil, nutmeg, parsley, sage, and thyme.

Benefits of the DASH Diet

Now that we have discussed what the DASH Diet is and since you have an overview already lets go to its health benefits. The DASH diet comes with a range of health benefits. Following are some of the major advantages of following the DASH diet:

Cardiovascular Health

The DASH diet decreases your consumption of refined carbohydrates by increasing your consumption of foods high in potassium and dietary fiber (fruits, vegetables, and whole grains). In addition, it diminishes your consumption of saturated fats. Therefore, the DASH diet has a favorable effect on your lipid profile and glucose tolerance, which reduces the prevalence of metabolic syndrome (MS) in post-menopausal women.

Reports state that a diet limited to 500 calories favors a loss of 17% of total body weight in 6 months in overweight women. This reduces the prevalence of MS by 15%. However, when this diet follows the patterns of the DASH diet, while triglycerides decrease in a similar way, the reduction in weight and BP is even greater.

It also reduces blood sugar and increases HDL, which decreases the prevalence of MS in 35% of women. These results contrast with those of other studies, which have reported that the DASH diet alone, i.e., without caloric restriction, does not affect HDL and glycemia. This means that the effects of the DASH diet on MS are associated mainly with the greater reduction in BP and that, for more changes, the diet would be required to be combined with weight loss.

Helpful for Patients with Diabetes

The DASH diet has also been shown to help reduce inflammatory and coagulation factors (C-reactive protein and fibrinogen) in patients with diabetes. These benefits are associated with the contribution of antioxidants and fibers, given the high consumption of fruits and vegetables that the DASH diet requires. In addition, the DASH diet has been shown to reduce total cholesterol and LDL, which reduces the estimated 10-year cardiovascular risk. Epidemiological studies have determined that women in the highest quintile of food consumption according to the DASH diet have a 24% to 33% lower risk of coronary events and an 18% lower risk of a cerebrovascular event. Similarly, a meta-analysis of six observational studies has determined that the DASH diet can reduce the risk of cardiovascular events by 20%.

Weight Reduction

Limited research associates the DASH diet, in isolation, with weight reduction. In some studies, weight reduction was greater when the subject was on the DASH diet as compared to an isocaloric controlled diet. This could be related to the higher calcium intake and lower energy density of the DASH diet. The American guidelines for the treatment of obesity emphasize that, regardless of diet, a caloric restriction would be the most important factor in reducing weight.

However, several studies have made an association between (1) greater weight and fat loss in diets and (2) caloric restriction and higher calcium intake. Studies have also observed an inverse association between dairy consumption and body mass index (BMI). In obese patients, weight loss has been reported as being 170% higher after 24 weeks on a hypocaloric diet with high calcium intake.

In addition, the loss of trunk fat was reported to be 34% of the total weight loss as compared to only 21% in a control diet. It has also been determined that a calcium intake of 20 mg per gram has a protective effect in overweight middle-aged women. This would be equivalent to 1275 mg of calcium for a western diet of 1700 kcal. It has been suggested that low calcium intake increases the circulating level of the parathyroid hormone and vitamin D, which have been shown to increase the level of cytosolic calcium in adipocytes in vitro, changing the metabolism of lipolysis to lipogenesis.

Despite these reports, the effect that diet-provided calcium has on women's weight after menopause is a controversial subject. An epidemiological study has noted that a sedentary lifestyle and, to a lesser extent, caloric intake are associated with post- menopausal weight gain, though calcium intake is not associated with it. The average calcium intake in this group of women is approximately 1000 mg, which would be low, as previously stated. Another study of post-menopausal women shows that calcium and vitamin D supplementation in those with a calcium intake of less than 1200 mg per day decreases the risk of weight gain by 11%.

In short, the DASH diet is favorable, both in weight control and in the regulation of fatty tissue deposits, due to its high calcium content (1200 mg/day). The contribution of calcium apparently plays a vital role in the regulation of lipogenesis.

Now that we have established the myriad benefits of the DASH diet, let's check out some of the most delicious and unique DASH diet recipes for all times of the day!

Importance of Healthy Weight

When we think of losing our excess weight, we often wonder what goal to set. But it is ideal to set 6 pounds as the weight loss goal and you have to lose it in 10 weeks. Here are some tips to bear in mind when you wish to do so.

• The very first tip is to eat a bowl of vegetables with each and every meal. Pick the best and freshest ones and don't season it with any salt or pepper. You can try a different color vegetable and steam it. If it is a soft vegetable then try to have it raw. You will see that your body is getting healthier with each meal and your palette will get used to eating vegetables on a regular basis.

• You must consume half a cup or bowl of nuts and seeds on a daily basis. You can have it twice if your palette allows it or stick to just one cup per day. You must not consume the salted variety and can prepare it at home with ease. Place 1 cup almond, 1-cup cashews and 1 cup unsalted pistachios in a pan and dry roast it. Allow it to cool down and place in an airtight container. You must eat at least half cup of this on a regular basis.

• You should limit your consumption of fatty meats. You have to remove the skin from your meats in order to make them diet friendly. You should also avoid the meats that are slightly salty like fish. You should clean the meats externally and cook it well in order to get rid of the sodium content. If you wish to use broth to cook it then you should use only homemade broth that is free from sodium.

• You should avoid dairy and soya product at least for the first 4 weeks of the diet. These have the tendency of increasing your body's fat content. If you are too used to these then you can replace them with nut extracts such as nut milk and nut yogurt. But you should limit these as well and have them in measured quantities.

• You have to cut out junk and processed foods from your diet at all costs. They have the tendency of filling up your body with all unnecessary chemicals that can make you extremely unhealthy. Try to come up with healthier versions of the diet.

•You have to drink at least 10 to 12 glasses of water a day. You can fill up a few bottles and label them. As soon as you finish the first bottle move to the next and then to the next etc.

•You have to exercise at least 40 minutes a day. The first 20 minutes should be hardcore cardio and the rest can be weights or floor exercises. You have to keep it as diverse as possible. Try to exercise at least 4 days a week.

•You might have to consume a few supplements that are laden with vitamins and minerals when you are following such a diet and exercise regime. You should consult a dietician for it and he or she might give you the appropriate advice.

These form the different things that you should do when you wish to lose this type of weight in 10 weeks. You have to buy yourself a quality weighing scale and weigh yourself from time to time in order to see if you are on the right track.

Why The DASH Diet Promotes Fast Weight Loss?

In addition to all its other health benefits, the DASH diet supports healthy weight loss. This is one of the major reasons for its popularity. Although the DASH diet wasn't formulated primarily for weight loss, such as the Atkins and Paleo diets, among others, if accompanied by an exercise routine, it can facilitate quick and healthy weight loss.

The advantage of the DASH diet is that it helps in weight loss and simultaneously aims towards overall healthiness. It encompasses a systematic approach towards food intake, focusing on certain food choices that aid weight loss while avoiding foods that lead to weight gain. It can also help wean oneself off blood pressure and diabetes medications.

The DASH diet includes lots of vegetables and fruits in its meal plans. Fruits and vegetables are typically low in calories, high in fiber, and are satiating. A weight loss drink or supplement can help you lose weight; however, it will not satiate your hunger. Therefore you are likely to eat more frequently, so your calorie intake will go up.

The diet includes certain protein rich-foods at each meal orsnack that are likewise filling, avoiding either in-between meals or blood sugar crashes due to a sudden spike of insulin.

The meal plans of the DASH diet are not overloaded with carbohydrates. The plans are generally low on starchy foods, instead including protein rich-foods that prevent muscle breakdown and boost the metabolism for faster weight loss.

Should you need more information than is contained here, there is a plethora of books, articles and journals available online that can provide additional plans and menus. If followed rigorously, they can help you achieve your desired results.

Health Benefits of Consuming Good Fats

The DASH diet comes with a range of health benefits. Following are some of the major advantages of following the DASH diet:

Cardiovascular Health

The DASH diet decreases your consumption of refined carbohydrates by increasing your consumption of foods high in potassium and dietary fiber (fruits, vegetables, and whole grains). In addition, it diminishes your consumption of saturated fats. Therefore, the DASH diet has a favorable effect on your lipid profile and glucose tolerance, which reduces the prevalence of metabolic syndrome (MS) in post-menopausal women.

Reports state that a diet limited to 500 calories favors a loss of 17% of total body weight in 6 months in overweight women. This reduces the prevalence of MS by 15%. However, when this diet follows the patterns of the DASH diet, while triglycerides decrease in a similar way, the reduction in weight and BP is even greater.

It also reduces blood sugar and increases HDL, which decreases the prevalence of MS in 35% of women. These results contrast with those of other studies, which have reported that the DASH diet alone, i.e., without caloric restriction, does not affect HDL and glycemia. This means that the effects of the DASH diet on MS are associated mainly with the greater reduction in BP and that, for more changes, the diet would be required to be combined with weight loss.

Helpful for Patients with Diabetes

The DASH diet has also been shown to help reduce inflammatory and coagulation factors (C-reactive protein and fibrinogen) in patients with diabetes. These benefits are associated with the contribution of antioxidants and fibers, given the high consumption of fruits and vegetables that the DASH diet requires. In addition, the DASH diet has been shown to reduce total cholesterol and LDL, which reduces the estimated 10-year cardiovascular risk. Epidemiological studies have determined that women in the highest quintile of food consumption according to the DASH diet have a 24% to 33% lower risk of coronary events and an 18% lower risk of a cerebrovascular event. Similarly, a meta-analysis of six observational studies has determined that the DASH diet can reduce the risk of cardiovascular events by 20%.

Weight Reduction

Limited research associates the DASH diet, in isolation, with weight reduction. In some studies, weight reduction was greater when the subject was on the DASH diet as compared to an isocaloric controlled diet. This could be related to the higher calcium intake and lower energy density of the DASH diet. The American guidelines for the treatment of obesity emphasize that, regardless of diet, a caloric restriction would be the most important factor in reducing weight.

However, several studies have made an association between (1) greater weight and fat loss in diets and (2) caloric restriction and higher calcium intake. Studies have also observed an inverse association between dairy consumption and body mass index (BMI). In obese patients, weight loss has been reported as being 170% higher after 24 weeks on a hypocaloric diet with high calcium intake.

In addition, the loss of trunk fat was reported to be 34% of the total weight loss as compared to only 21% in a control diet. It has also been determined that a calcium intake of 20 mg per gram has a protective effect in overweight middle-aged women. This would be equivalent to 1275 mg of calcium for a western diet of 1700 kcal. It has been suggested that low calcium intake increases the circulating level of the parathyroid hormone and vitamin D, which have been shown to increase the level of cytosolic calcium in adipocytes in vitro, changing the metabolism of lipolysis to lipogenesis.

Despite these reports, the effect that diet-provided calcium has on women's weight after menopause is a controversial subject. An epidemiological study has noted that a sedentary lifestyle and, to a lesser extent, caloric intake are associated with post-menopausal weight gain, though calcium intake is not associated with it. The average calcium intake in this group of women is approximately 1000 mg, which would be low, as previously stated. Another study of post-menopausal women shows that calcium and vitamin D supplementation in those with a calcium intake of less than 1200 mg per day decreases the risk of weight gain by 11%.

In short, the DASH diet is favorable, both in weight control and in the regulation of fatty tissue deposits, due to its high calcium content (1200 mg/day). The contribution of calcium apparently plays a vital role in the regulation of lipogenesis.

Now that we have established the myriad benefits of the DASH diet, let's check out some of the most delicious and unique DASH diet recipes for all times of the day!

Dash Food Groups Intake

All the DASH plans follow roughly this balance between the groups.

Grains:

The only source of processed food in DASH is grains, but these must be whole grains to conform to the diet. The reason for this is that they are higher in fiber and have less of an effect on blood sugar. Whole grain, steel-cut, and unbleached are what to look for on the label. Cereals, pasta, breads, and rice are all sources of grains but some are more processed than others. For example, granola is often less processed than a corn puff cereal. You can also try other grain substitutes like quinoa which also has a high protein content. A good rule is to stay away from any packaged food that looks white. White pasta, white bread, white flour etc., have all been refined and processed so they are essentially empty calories with no useful nutrition.

Vegetables:

Not all vegetables are created equal. Aim to buy fresh or frozen rather than tinned as these tend to be loaded with added sodium. Avoid any that come with sauces or added salt. Vegetables are a large part of DASH because your body needs fiber and vitamins but also because they are lower in calories. Some vegetables are not allowed on DASH because they cause high blood sugar spikes or are not nutritional enough. White potatoes are a prime example of this because they are heavy with starch which is then metabolized into pure sugar. Your body naturally metabolizes starches into sugars so you could be eating a sugary diet without even realizing it. Cruciferous greens and leafy greens are all advised on DASH as well as eating a colorful variety when possible.

Some vegetables, like beans, are actually legumes. These are perfect for DASH because they are high in protein and fiber without being animal products or being processed. If you're using canned beans look for low sodium and rinse them before use.

Dairy:

While many think that dairy is part of getting enough protein it's actually rather unnecessary. Swapping dairy for nut products is a good approach for DASH followers where possible. Dairy is allowed on DASH as long as it is low-fat with no added sugar. Many dairy products that are low-fat are pumped up with processed sugar to improve the taste. This means that even though the fat number is lower the calorie number is higher from the sugar. Yogurt is a prime example of this. Dairy can be a very filling choice, and it's also a supplemented source of vitamins D, B and A. Always read the ingredients on dairy products and avoid any with added hormones.

Fruits:

While fruits often get lumped together with vegetables, the DASH approach keeps them separate because you have to limit your intake. Most fruits are high in sugars which means that they cause your blood sugar to rise quickly. These are not allowed at all during phase one and only in a limited quantity during phase two. Despite the fact that fruits are often full of nutrients and fiber the amount they have does not balance out the huge levels of fructose and other natural sugars. Many processed fruits also have added sugar, making this worse. Dried and canned fruits are a prime example of this and should be avoided entirely. Fruit juice is also not recommended as it is literally a refined sugar cocktail.

Nuts & Seeds

These can be the perfect snacking item as they are rich in healthy fats and fiber. The problem with many nuts is that they are salted. This makes them wholly unsuitable for DASH. You'll also need to be careful with the serving size as they tend to be very calorie dense foods. Nut butters are a great alternative to sugary jams and an ideal snack food to include on DASH. Consider making your own or looking in the natural food section if you can't find ones without additives. Peanut butter can be especially problematic as many companies add xylitol to improve taste.

Animal Products

As you've seen it's important to limit animal products on DASH. Animals products like meat, eggs, and dairy all contain high amounts of cholesterol and saturated fat which is why they should be eaten in moderation only. Look for leaner cuts and grass-fed products where possible. A serving of any animal product should be limited to 3oz, this includes seafood. Avoid processed meat products like ham as they are pumped up with added salt to improve the flavor and help with preservation. It's a good idea to look at buying a slicer or making extra at dinner time so you can slice home cooked meats as "deli" leftovers instead which you know do not have added salt.

Fats

While not technically a food group fat are often added to foods to improve the taste or we use them to cook. Foods that are labeled as "fat-free" are often nothing more than a marketing ploy and may be loaded with sugar and much higher in calories. Your body and brain need fat to function so choosing unsaturated fats like avocado oil or coconut oil over more refined (canola) or animal fats (lard) is a much better choice. You can use grass fed butter for cooking as long as you include it in your daily allowance of animal products, the same goes for ghee. Avoid products that are heavily processed such as vegetable oils, margarine, shortening, frying oils and any that contain trans fats. Most trans-fats are difficult for the body to process and consuming them has been strongly linked to weight gain.

Enhance your Results with Exercise

We all know that exercise is healthy but is it absolutely necessary in order to benefit from the DASH diet? Contrary to what many health advocates will tell you, going out of your way to exercise is not necessary for everyone. It depends on your own unique lifestyle. If you are a very active person or have a job that requires you to do a lot of manual labor, then chances are that you don't need to go out of your way to exercise. For example, if you work construction then going out of your way to exercise would be a bit repetitive since you get enough exercise working. However, if you work behind a desk then you probably need to take proactive steps to exercise.

The truth is that exercising, in combination with a healthy diet, will give you more energy and make you feel so much better! There are a lot of benefits to exercising that we're going to look at but just remember that you should always take things slowly. Don't start intense workouts immediately. You will need to work your way into it slowly.

Exercise Helps Control Weight

Exercise will help you control your weight because of its powerful impact on your metabolism. You'll prevent excess weight gain while also making it easier to lose weight in the first place. The truth is that while exercise is not a requirement in weight loss, it does make it so much easier.

You will burn calories when active. The more intense the activity, the more calories you will burn. While regular trips to the gym are highly beneficial, some people just can't afford to invest in the time required to be consistent so my advice is to find ways to become more active that fit into your everyday life. I will walk through a number of these methods later in the book.

Exercise Combats Disease and Other Health Conditions

DASH dieting is designed to help prevent high blood pressure so it's worth noting that exercise can actually enhance its effect. Exercise will also help prevent high blood pressure while also boosting your immune system. Furthermore, being active will boost your high-density lipoprotein (HDL) cholesterol which is also known as "good cholesterol." It also lowers those unhealthy triglycerides, known as "bad cholesterol."

Most doctors who prescribe DASH dieting will also encourage patients to exercise regularly. It's a powerful one-two punch!

Being active will also help prevent other health issues like stroke, metabolic syndrome, and even diabetes.

Exercise Improves your Mood

If you find yourself needing an emotional lift then you need look no further than exercise. A short session in the gym or a 30-minute walk will improve your mood. When you're physically active, a number of chemicals are released in the brain. These chemicals will make you happier and more relaxed.

Furthermore, exercise will help you feel better about your appearance so it boosts your confidence. Self-esteem is an important part of any lifestyle change. When you start growing confident in yourself, it becomes easier to stay consistent. You'll work harder on these improvements.

Exercise is the Best Energy Booster!

You might wonder how being physically active will actually give you more energy. After all, exercising results in fatigue – at least that's what most people believe. Regular activity will provide a boost to your muscle growth, therefore giving you a significant metabolic boost. That's why we tend to have more energy after a big workout.

Exercising allows your tissues to soak in oxygen, which improves your blood flow. In short, it gives you much more energy throughout the day. That's why exercising in the morning is so beneficial.

Exercise will Help you Sleep Better

If you are having trouble sleeping at night, then exercise is a solution! It helps you fall asleep faster and will even deepen your sleep. That's why people who have active jobs tend to get better sleep. Their schedule is consistent because they have no trouble falling asleep. They feel better and wake up earlier.

However, just make sure that you don't exercise too close to your bedtime. You will be too energized to fall asleep. Instead, an evening session should take place at least 4 hours prior to bed time.

Exercise is a Fun and Social Experience

There are a number of ways that you can enjoy the benefits of physical activity, many of which are quite enjoyable. So, don't limit yourself to spending hours on the treadmill or walking the same route every day. Try to engage in activities that you enjoy. Sports are a great way to get in your exercise while having a blast! Dance lessons are another!

Find activities that make you happy. That way you will be more likely to consistently follow through with them. If you get bored, then try something new.

How Often Should You Exercise?

First of all, you so not have to go out of your way to becoming more active. There are several ways that you can become more active. We're about to look at some of them, but for now just understand that you will need to aim for at least 100 minutes of moderate activity every week.

Try to make small changes so that your body has a chance to adapt and then slightly increase your activity until you hit your final goal. I do encourage at least two 30-minute weight training sessions per week since building your muscle mass provides you with a permanent metabolic boost. In other words, the more muscles you have, the more calories your body will burn throughout the day.

Simple Ways to Become More Active

It's easy to get swept away by our everyday lives. We call it "fast-paced" but for many, this life of all work and no play is mostly sitting behind a desk. While it is definitely busy work-wise, it's not exactly an active lifestyle. That's why it's important to take steps to add physical activity into our everyday life.

The following methods are an easy way to become more active in your everyday life. You'll start to become more mindful about these little things and turn everyday tasks into mini-workouts. You will be amazed at how much better you feel.

Walk More

Rather than driving two blocks to pick up the latest magazine from the magazine stand, walk those two blocks. This one simple decision will get you a 10-15-minute workout without having to go out of your way. You can also go for walks while chatting with your friend. Whatever it takes to walk more rather than just sitting around will help you become more active.

Take the Stairs Rather than the Elevator

Did you know that just five minutes of walking up the stairs can burn as many as 150 calories? If you work on an upper floor, then start walking up the stairs rather than taking the elevator. This is a small change where you don't really have to go out of your way to become more active. If you do these five times per week you have the potential to burn over 700 calories!

Clean More

Not only is having a clean house an amazing feeling, cleaning can burn up to 200 calories an hour. You should clean for at least one hour per week. Having a clean home is motivational and you will be killing two birds with one stone. Your home will be clean and you'll be burning 200 calories every week with no extra effort.

Use a Basket for Shopping Whenever Possible

If you are just making a short trip into the store, then you should use a basket rather than a cart. It's automatic for us to reach for a cart no matter what but when you use a basket, you're getting in an automatic weightlifting session. It can actually add up to quite the workout.

Park Further Away

While everyone else is fighting tooth and nail for those close parking spots, start parking further away so that you are forced to walk further. You will actually save a lot of time that you would have wasted looking for a close parking spot. Additionally, you will get in a mini workout by walking further.

Start Playing with your Pet

It goes without saying but if you have a dog, then you will have to go on frequent walks. So why not take it a step further by playing with your furry friend. Dogs are full of energy and will happily play games. You can get in a good workout while your dog stays happy! You can do the same thing with your cat. They also love to play but you'll usually have to initiate it. My point is that playing with your pet is an amazingly fun way to stay active.

Get Up At Least Once Every Hour

It's easy to lose track of time while working behind a desk so set an alarm to remind yourself to get up every hour. You should walk around or stretch for a minimum of two minutes before returning to your work. There are also programs like Break Pal that not only alert you when it's time to stand, but they give you a few simple tasks to perform before sitting back down.

The point that I am trying to make here is that small additions to your routine can make a huge difference. These changes will make it so that you don't have to go out of your way to exercise to become more active. Once you establish new habits, they become an automatic part of your everyday routine.

Exercises to Enhance the DASH Diet

For those of you who want to enhance the DASH diet even further, then you will want to include a few exercises into your daily routine. We'll look at some of the best workouts to include while DASH dieting.

Aerobic Exercise

Aerobic exercises will improve your circulation and help lower your blood pressure, making them the absolute best form of exercise to combine with DASH dieting. Additionally, it will help control how strongly your heart pumps blood and reduce the risk of type-2 diabetes. Even if you already have diabetes, aerobic exercise will help your body control glucose levels.

Frequency: You should aim to exercise at least 120 minutes per week.

Examples of Aerobic Exercise

- Walking
- Running
- Swimming
- Cycling
- Sports
- Jump Rope

Strength Training

Strength training will have a more specific effect on the composition of your body. Individuals who are hauling around a lot of excess fat will find strength training to be quite beneficial to their weight loss efforts. Additionally, studies have shown that the combination of aerobic exercise and strength training actually lowers bad cholesterol levels while raising good cholesterol levels.

Frequency: Strength training workouts should be performed at least two days a week, making sure to rest for at least one day in between.

Examples of Strength Training Exercises

- Weightlifting
- Curling
- Resistance band workouts
- Push-ups
- Squats
- Pull-ups

Breakfast Recipes

Sweet Avocado Smoothie

Preparation Time: 5 minutes | Cooking Time: 0 minutes | Servings: 2

Ingredients:

2 Cups Ice Cubes

1 Teaspoon Vanilla Extract, Pure

1 ½ Teaspoons Granulated Stevia 1 ½ Cups Milk, Nonfat

1 ½ Cups Peaches, Frozen

1 Cup Vanilla Greek Yogurt

1 Tablespoon Flaxseed, Ground

1 Avocado, Peeled & Pitted

Directions:

Blend all ingredients until smooth, and serve chilled.

Nutrition:

Calories: 323 Protein: 21 Grams Fat: 15 Grams, Carbs: 32 Grams, Sodium: 142 mg Cholesterol: 9 mg

Cinnamon Apple Overnight Oats

Preparation Time: 8 hours and 15 minutes | Cooking Time: 0 minutes | Servings: 2

Ingredients:

1 Cup Old Fashioned Rolled Oats

2 Tablespoons Chia Seeds - 1 ¼ Cup Milk, Nonfat

½ Tablespoon Ground Cinnamon

2 Teaspoons Honey, Raw

½ Teaspoon Vanilla Extract, Pure

Dash Sea Salt

1 Apple, Diced

Directions:

Divide your chia seeds, oats, cinnamon, milk, honey, vanilla, and salt in mason jars. Place the lids on, and shake well until thoroughly combined. Remove the lids, and then add half of your diced apples to each jar. Sprinkle with cinnamon. Put the lids tightly back on the jars, and refrigerate overnight.

Nutrition:

Calories: 339 Protein: 13 Grams Fat: 8 Grams, Carbs: 60 Grams Sodium: 66 mg Cholesterol: 3 mg

Blueberry Muffins

Preparation Time: 20 minutes

Cooking Time: 25 minutes

Servings: 12

Ingredients:

1 ¼ Cup Whole Wheat Flour

½ Cup Old Fashioned Rolled Oats

1 Teaspoon Baking Soda

1 Teaspoon Baking Powder

¼ Teaspoon Ground Cinnamon

¼ Teaspoon Sea Salt, Fine

¼ Cup Olive Oil

¼ Cup Dark Brown Sugar

1 Teaspoon Vanilla Extract, Pure

2 Eggs, Large

2/3 Cup Milk

1 Cup Blueberries, Fresh or Frozen

8 Medjool Dates, Pitted & Chopped

Directions:

Start by heating your oven to 350, and then line a muffin tin with liners.

Get out a bowl and stir your oats, flour, baking soda, baking powder, cinnamon and salt together until well combined.

Get out a different bowl and whisk your olive oil and brown sugar until the mixture turns fluffy. Whisk in the eggs one egg at a time until it's well beaten, and then add in your milk and vanilla extract. Beat to combine.

Pour your flour mixture with your wet ingredients, mixing well. Evenly spoon the batter between your muffin cups, and bake for twenty-five minutes. Allow to cool before storing.

Nutrition:

Calories: 180, Protein: 4 Grams, Fat: 6 Grams, Carbs: 30 Grams, Sodium: 172 mg, Cholesterol: 35 mg

Yogurt & Banana Muffins

Preparation Time: 15 minutes | Cooking Time: 25 minutes | Servings: 4

Ingredients:

3 Bananas, Large & Mashed

1 Teaspoon Baking Soda - 1 Cup Old Fashioned Rolled Oats

2 Tablespoons Flaxseed, Ground - 1 Cup Whole Wheat Flour

¼ Cup Applesauce, Unsweetened - ½ Cup Plain Yogurt

¼ Cup Brown Sugar - 2 Teaspoons Vanilla Extract, Pure

Directions:

Start by turning the oven to 355, and then get out a muffin tray. Grease it and then get out a bowl. Mix your flaxseed, oats, soda, and flour in a bowl. Mash your banana and then mix in your sugar, vanilla, yogurt and applesauce. Stir in your oats mixture, making sure it's well combined. It's okay for it to be lumpy. Divide between muffin trays, and then bake for twenty-five minutes. Serve warm.

Nutrition:

Calories: 316 Protein: 11.2 Grams Fat: 14.5 Grams, Carbs: 36.8 Grams Sodium: 469 mg Cholesterol: 43 mg

Berry Quinoa Bowls

Preparation Time: 15 minutes | Cooking Time: 20 minutes | Servings: 2

Ingredients:

1 Small Peach, Sliced

2/3 + ¾ Cup Milk, Low Fat

1/3 Cup Uncooked Quinoa, Rinsed Well

½ Teaspoon Vanilla Extract, Pure

2 Teaspoons Brown Sugar - 14 Blueberries

2 Teaspoons Honey, Raw

12 Raspberries

Directions:

Start to boil your quinoa, vanilla, 2/3 cup milk and brown sugar together for five minutes before reducing it to a simmer. Cook for twenty minutes. Heat a grill pan that's been greased over medium heat, and then add in your peaches to grill for one minute per side. Heat the remaining ¾ cup of milk in your microwave. Cook the quinoa with a splash of milk, berries and grilled peaches. Don't forget to drizzle with honey before serving it.

Nutrition:

Calories: 435 Protein: 9.2 Grams Fat: 13.7 Grams, Carbs: 24.9 Grams Sodium: 141 m, Cholesterol: 78 mg

Pineapple Green Smoothie

Preparation Time: 5 minutes | Cooking Time: 0 minutes | Servings: 2

Ingredients:

1 ¼ Cups Orange Juice

½ Cup Greek Yogurt, Plain

1 Cup Spinach, Fresh

1 Cup Pineapple, Frozen & Chunked

1 Cup Mango, Frozen & Chunked

1 Tablespoons Ground Flaxseed

1 Teaspoon Granulated Stevia

Directions:

Start by blending everything together until smooth, and then serve cold.

Nutrition:

Calories: 213, Protein: 9 Grams Fat: 2, Grams Carbs: 43 Grams, Sodium: 44 mg, Cholesterol: 2.5 mg

Peanut Butter & Banana Smoothie

Preparation Time: 5 minutes | Cooking Time: 0 minutes | Servings: 1

Ingredients:

1 Cup Milk, Nonfat

1 Tablespoons Peanut Butter, All Natural

1 Banana, Frozen & Sliced

Directions:

Start by blending everything together until smooth.

Nutrition:

Calories: 146, Protein: 1.1 Grams, Fat: 5.5 Grams, Carbs: 1.8 Grams

Mushroom Frittata

Preparation Time: 15 minutes| Cooking Time: 10 minutes | Servings: 4

Ingredients:

4 Shallots, Chopped - 1 Tablespoons Butter

2 Teaspoons parsley, Fresh & Diced - ½ lb. Mushrooms, Fresh & Diced - 3 Eggs

1 Teaspoon Thyme - 5 Egg Whites

¼ Teaspoon Black Pepper

1 Tablespoon Half & Half, Fat Free - ¼ Cup Parmesan Cheese, Grated

Directions:

Start by turning the oven to 350, and then get out a skillet. Grease it with butter, letting it melt over medium heat. Once your butter is hot adding in your shallots. Cook until golden brown, which should take roughly five minutes. Stir in your thyme, pepper, parsley and mushrooms. Beat your eggs, egg whites, parmesan, and half and half together in a bowl. Pour the mixture over your mushrooms, cooking for two minutes. Transfer the skillet to the oven, and bake for fifteen minutes. Slice to serve warm.

Nutrition:

Calories: 391 Protein: 7.6 Grams Fat: 12.8 Grams, Carbs: 31.5 Grams Sodium: 32 mg, Cholesterol: 112 mg

Cheesy Omelet

Preparation Time: 10 minutes | Cooking Time: 10 minutes | Servings: 4

Ingredients:

4 Eggs

4 Cups Broccoli Florets

1 Tablespoons Olive Oil

1 Cup Egg Whites

¼ Cup Cheddar, Reduced Fat

¼ Cup Romano, Grated

¼ Teaspoon Sea Salt, Fine

¼ Teaspoon Black Pepper

Cooking Spray as Needed

Directions:

Start by heating your oven to 350, and then steam your broccoli over boiling water for five to seven minutes. It should be tender.

Mash the broccoli into small pieces, and then toss with salt, pepper and olive oil.

Get out a muffin tray and then grease it with cooking spray. Divide your broccoli between the cups, and then get out a bowl.

In the bowl beat your eggs with salt, pepper, egg whites and parmesan.

Pour your batter over the broccoli, and then top with cheese. Bake for two minutes before serving warm.

Nutrition:

Calories: 427, Protein: 7.5 Grams, Fat: 8.6 Grams, Carbs: 13 Grams, Sodium: 282 mg, Cholesterol: 4.2 Grams

Ginger Congee

Preparation Time: 10 minutes | Cooking Time: 1 hour | Servings: 1

Ingredients:

1 Cup White Rice, Long Grain & Rinsed

7 Cups Chicken Stock

1 Inch Ginger, Peeled & Sliced Thin

Green Onion, Sliced for Garnish

Sesame Seed Oil to Garnish

Directions:

Start by boiling your ginger, rice and salt in a pot. Allow it to simmer and reduce to low heat. Give it a gentle stir, and then allow it to cook for an hour. It should be thick and creamy.

Garnish by drizzling with sesame oil and serving warm.

Nutrition:

Calories: 510, Protein: 13.5 Grams, Carbs: 60.7 Grams, Fat: 24.7 Grams Sodium: 840 mg, Cholesterol: 0 mg

Egg Melts

Preparation Time: 10 minutes | Cooking Time: 10 minutes | Servings: 2

Ingredients:

1 Teaspoon Olive oil

2 English Muffins, Whole Grain & Split

4 Scallions, Sliced Fine

8 Egg Whites, Whisked

¼ Teaspoon Sea Salt, Fine

¼ Teaspoon Black Pepper

½ Cup Swiss Cheese, Shredded & Reduced Fat

½ Cup Grape Tomatoes, Quartered

Directions:

Set the oven to broil, and then put your English muffins on a baking sheet. Make sure the split side is facing up. Broil for two minutes. They should turn golden around the edges.

Get out a skillet and grease with oil. Place it over medium heat, and cook your scallions for three minutes.

Beat your egg whites with salt and pepper, and pour this over your scallions.

Cook for another minute, stirring gently.

Spread this on your muffins, and top with remaining scallions if desired, cheese and tomatoes. Broil for 1 and a half more minutes to melt the cheese and serve warm.

Nutrition:

Calories: 212, Protein: 5.3 Grams, Fat: 3.9 Grams, Carbs: 14.3 Grams, Sodium: 135 mg, Cholesterol: 0 mg

Fluffy Pancakes for Breakfast

Preparation Time: 10 minutes | Cooking Time: 10 minutes | Servings: 2

Ingredients:

Eggs – 1

Melted butter – 2 tablespoons

White vinegar – 2 tablespoons

Milk – 3/4 cup

All-purpose flour – 1 cup

Baking powder – 1 teaspoon

Baking soda – 1/2 teaspoon

White sugar – 2 tablespoons

Salt – 1/2 teaspoon

Cooking spray

Directions:

Begin with mixing milk and vinegar in a bowl and leave the solution for 5 minutes until it turns "sour".

Whip egg and butter together into the "soured" milk emulsion.

Add all-purpose flour, baking powder, baking soda, sugar, and salt in a separate bowl.

Take all the wet component and mix with the flour emulsion. Whisk the mixture until it becomes an even paste.

Take a frying pan and heat it over medium heat. Now coat the pan with cooking spray.

Take 1/4 cupful of the paste in a frying pan and cook well. Use a spatula to flip the cake and cook until it turns fluffy and golden brown.

Transfer the pancakes onto a plate and garnish with your choice of cream.

Nutrition:

Proteins: 6.4 g, Carbohydrates: 32.7 g, Fat: 8.2 g

Fluffy Zucchini Bread

Preparation Time: 20 minutes | Cooking Time: 1 hour | Servings: 24

Ingredients:

All-purpose white flour – 3 cups

Salt – 1 teaspoon

Baking soda – 1 teaspoon

Baking powder – 1 teaspoon

Cinnamon (ground) – – 1 teaspoon

Eggs – 3

Vegetable oil – 1 cup

Sugar – 2 1/4 cups

Vanilla extract – 3 teaspoons

Zucchini (grated) – 2 cups

Walnuts (chopped) – 1 cup

Directions:

Start by preheating the oven to 325 degrees F (165 degrees C).

Now grease two 9 x 5-inch pans or standard pans with cooking oil.

Flour the greased pans and remove the access flour.

Mix flour along with salt, baking powder, baking soda, and ground cinnamon.

In a separate bowl, take eggs, vegetable oil, sugar and vanilla extract and beat all the ingredients together.

Add dry flour mixture in the creamed solution and beat until it becomes a thick paste.

Grate two cups of zucchini.

Add grated zucchini and chopped walnuts in the paste and stir until all the ingredients are well combined in the flour paste.

Now pour the batter into the greased pans and bake for at least 40 to 60 minutes. Use a tester if required.

Let the bread cool in the pan until it is firm enough to be removed.

Cut into slices once the bread is completely cool.

Keep the remaining in the refrigerator.

Nutrition:

Proteins: 3.3 g, Carbohydrates: 32.1 g, Fat: 13.1 g

Spinach Crustless Quiche

Preparation Time: 20 minutes | Cooking Time: 30 minutes | Servings: 6

Ingredients:

Vegetable oil – 1 tablespoon

Chopped onion – 1

Frozen chopped spinach – 10 ounce/1 package

Eggs – 5

Muenster cheese (shredded) – 3 cups

Salt – 1/4 teaspoon

Black pepper (ground) – 1/8 teaspoon

Directions:

Begin with preheating the oven to 350 degrees F (175 degrees C).

Now grease a 9 x 5 inch pan or any standard pan with cooking oil.

Chop the onion and remove the frozen spinach in a strainer. Squeeze spinach to remove all the extra moisture or water.

Heat vegetable oil in a large frying pan and add chopped onion into it. Cook onions until they turn soft or light golden in color.

Add drained spinach into it and stir until moisture gets evaporated and remover the mixture.

Take eggs in a fresh bowl and whip. Add salt, cheese, and pepper into it.

Now take the spinach mixture and add to the whipped egg solution and stir until everything is blended well.

Pour mixture into the greased pan and bake in the oven for 30 minutes.

Leave the dish until it cools and serve by cutting into slices of your choice

Nutrition:

Proteins: 20.4 g, Carbohydrates: 4.8 g, Fat: 23.7 g

Friendly French Toast

Preparation Time: 10 minutes | Cooking Time: 20 minutes | Servings: 12

Ingredients:

All-purpose flour – 1/4 cup

Milk – 1 cup

Salt – 1/2 teaspoon

Eggs – 3

Cinnamon (ground)– 1/2 teaspoon

Vanilla extract – 1 teaspoon

Sugar – 1 tablespoon

Bread – 12 slices

Directions: Take all-purpose flour in a bowl and add milk, eggs, salt (as per taste) and ground cinnamon, vanilla extract, and sugar. Whisk the mixture to make a smooth paste. Take a frying pan and heat it lightly. Take a slice of bread and soak it completely in the paste. Repeat this with all the slices. Now cook each slice of bread until it turns golden brown on both sides. Serve hot with maple syrup.

Nutrition:

Proteins: 4.8 g, Carbohydrates: 19.4 g, Fat: 2.7 g

Everyday Crepes

Preparation Time: 10 minutes | Cooking Time: 20 minutes | Servings: 4

Ingredients:

All-purpose flour – 1 cup

Eggs – 2

Milk – 1/2 cup

Water – 1/2 cup

Salt – 1/4 teaspoon

Butter (melted) – 2 tablespoons

Directions:

Start by taking all-purpose flour in a mixing bowl and or milk, water, salt, eggs and whisk together to make a running paste.

Add melted butter to the paste.

Heat a frying pan on medium flame and add a quarter cup of the batter into it.

Spread the batter evenly in the frying pan and let the crepe cook on both the sides. Serve hot.

Nutrition:

Proteins: 7.4 g   Carbohydrates: 25.5 g   Fat: 9.2 g

Hash Brown Cheesy Ham Casserole

Preparation Time: 15 minutes | Cooking Time: 1 hour | Servings: 12

Ingredients:

Hash brown potatoes (frozen package) – 1

Diced ham (cooked) – 8 ounces

Cream of potato soup (condensed) – 2 cans

Sour cream – 1

Cheddar cheese (shredded) – 2 cups

Parmesan cheese (grated) – 1 1/2 cups

Directions:

Start by preheating the oven to 375 degrees F (190 degrees C).

In a fresh bowl, take frozen packaged mix hash browns potatoes, diced cooked ham, shredded cheddar cheese, sour cream, and condensed cream of potato soup. Mix all the ingredients evenly. Now grease a large 9x13 inch baking dish and spread the mixture into it. Sprinkle grated parmesan cheese to cover the mixture evenly in the baking dish. Bake the dish in the oven for an hour until it is light brown in color. Serve hot garnished with parmesan cheese

Nutrition:

Proteins: 14.4 g, Carbohydrates: 29.7 g, Fat: 27.2 g

Baffle Waffles

Preparation Time: 10 minutes | Cooking Time: 15 minutes | Servings: 5

Ingredients::

All-purpose flour – 2 cups

Salt – 1 teaspoon

Baking powder – 4 teaspoons

Sugar – 2 tablespoons

Eggs – 2

Milk (warm) – 1 1/2 cups

Butter (melted) – 1/3 cup

Vanilla extract – 1 teaspoon

Directions:

Start by preheating the waffle iron to your desired set temperature.

Now take a fresh large bowl and add two cups of all-purpose flour, one teaspoon of salt, four teaspoons of baking powder and two teaspoons of sugar.

Stir all the ingredients in the mixture together and keep it aside.

Now take a third of a cup of butter and melt it.

Now in a fresh bowl take two eggs and mix with warm milk, melted butter and one teaspoon of vanilla extract.

Empty the mixture into the flour mixture and whisk it well to create a slurpy batter.

Now grease the preheated waffle iron and pour the batter evenly on it.

Close the waffle iron and cook until waffles turn crispy golden.

Top the waffle with whipped cream, maple syrup or fruit of your choice and serve hot.

Nutrition:

Proteins: 10.2 g, Carbohydrates: 47.6, Fat: 16.2

Banana Sour Cream Bread

Preparation Time: 10 minutes | Cooking Time: 1 hour | Servings: 32

Ingredients:

Sugar – 3 cups

Cinnamon (ground) – 1 teaspoon

Butter – 3/4 cup

Eggs – 3

Ripe bananas (mashed) – 6

Sour cream – 1 container

Vanilla extract – 2 teaspoons

Cinnamon (ground) – 2 teaspoons

Salt – 1/2 teaspoon

Baking soda – 3 teaspoons

All-purpose flour – 4 1/2 cups

Chopped walnuts (optional) – 1 cup

Directions:

Start by preheating the oven to 300 degrees F (150 degrees C).

Take two large loaf pans and grease evenly

Take a small bowl and add 1/4 cup white sugar, 1 teaspoon ground cinnamon and stir them together.

Now take the cinnamon and sugar mixture and dust spray the greased loaf pans.

Take a fresh bowl and add ripe bananas to mash well.

In a separate bowl take 3/4 cup of butter and three cups of white sugar. Mix them well.

Add three eggs to the same bowl, mashed bananas and mix them well.

Now add 16 ounces of sour cream, and two teaspoons of vanilla extract and two teaspoons of ground cinnamon and stir it well.

Add half teaspoon of salt, three teaspoons baking soda and four cups of all-purpose flour to the bowl. Stir to make a paste. You can also add walnuts to the paste (Optional). Mix them well into the batter. Now evenly spread the batter in the greased large loaf pans and bake well for one hour.

Insert a toothpick in the center of the pans to check if the bread is baked properly. Cut into slices and serve. Put the remaining bread in the refrigerator.

Nutrition:

Proteins: 3.7 g, Carbohydrates: 40.1 g, Fat: 10.4 g

Cinnamon Baked Bread

Preparation Time: 15 minutes | Cooking Time: 35 minutes | Servings: 15

Ingredients:

Refrigerated biscuit dough – 3 packages

Sugar – 1 cup

Cinnamon (ground) – 2 teaspoons

Margarine – 1/2 cup

Brown sugar – 1 cup

Chopped walnuts (optional) – 1/2 cup

Raisins – 1/2 cup

Directions:

Start by preheating the oven to 350 degrees F (175 degrees C).

Take a hard surface 9-inch Bundt pan and grease well with cooking spray.

Now take a cup of sugar and two teaspoons of ground cinnamon in a resealable plastic bag. Mix them well together.

Take three packets of refrigerated biscuits dough and cut each dough piece into small quarters.

Add at least 8 chopped biscuit dough pieces in the sugar-cinnamon mixture.

Seal the plastic bag and shake well until the dough pieces get evenly coated in sugar-cinnamon mixture.

Put a layer of sugar-cinnamon coated pieces in the bottom of the greased Bundt pan.

You can also add chopped walnuts and raisins over the layer to get the crunchy flavor. This step is totally optional.

Continue with a layer of sugar-cinnamon dough in the Bundt pan.

Take a frying pan pour half a cup of margarine and a cup of brown sugar.

Cook the mixture until margarine is completely melted and mixed well with sugar to form a smooth thick paste. Let the mixture boil for two minutes.

Now evenly pour the mixture over the biscuit dough placed inside Bundt pan.

Bake the bread in the preheated oven (350 degrees F) for 35 minutes until it turns puffy and golden brown.

Remove the pan and let the bread cool in Bundt pan for at least 10 minutes.

Once cooled, flip the Bundt pan and remove the bread onto a plate.

Nutrition:

Proteins: 5.3 g Carbohydrates: 61.5 g Fat: 17.7 g

Buttermilk Pancake

Preparation Time: 15 minutes | Cooking Time: 10 minutes | Servings: 12

Ingredients:

All-purpose flour – 3 cups

White sugar – 3 tablespoons

Baking powder – 3 teaspoons

Baking soda – 1 1/2 teaspoons

Salt – 3/4 teaspoon

Buttermilk – 3 cups

Milk – 1/2 cup

Eggs – 3

Butter (melted) – 1/3 cup

Directions:

Begin with preheating the to 200 degrees F.

In a fresh bowl take three cups of all-purpose, three tablespoons of sugar, three teaspoons of baking powder, 1 1/2 teaspoons of baking soda, and 3/4 teaspoon salt and stir it well.

Take a fresh bowl and add three large eggs, three cups of buttermilk, 1/2 cup of milk, and 1/3 cup of butter and stir them well together.

Now empty the mixture in the flour mixture and mix well until the batter turns slightly lumpy. Avoid making it too thin or too thick.

Take a large frying pan and heat it on medium flame.

Brush the pan with the butter using a scapula.

Use half cup batter and pour over the hot pan. Turn the batter upside down with a spatula once each side is evenly golden brown in color.

Remove the cakes on a plate and transfer them in the preheated oven to stay warm.

Use the remaining batter to make cakes.

Once cooked, serve hit with maple syrup or spread of your choice.

Nutrition:

Proteins: 7.2 g, Carbohydrates: 30.7 g, Fat: 7.4 g

French Toast with Blueberries

Preparation Time: 15 minutes

Cooking Time: 1 hour and 15 minutes

Servings: 10

Ingredients:

Day-old bread – 12 slices

Cream cheese – 2 packages

Fresh blueberries – 1 cup

Eggs – 12

Milk – 2 cups

Vanilla extract – 1 teaspoon

Maple syrup – 1/3 cup

White sugar – 1 cup

Cornstarch – 2 tablespoons

Water – 1 cup

Blueberries – 1 cup

Butter– 1 tablespoon

Directions:

Take a 9x13 inch baking dish and evenly grease it with cooking spray.

Now cut 12 slices of day-old small bread into one-inch cube each.

Take half of the sliced bread cubes in the baking dish

Now cut two eight once of packages of creamed cheese into one-inch cubes and put them nicely over the layer of arranged bread cubes in the baking dish. Take one cup of fresh blueberries and sprinkle them over bread cubes on cream cheese. Top the blueberries with remaining pieces of bread cubes. Now take a fresh large bowl and break 12 eggs into it and beat nicely. Add two cups of milk, one teaspoon of vanilla extract and 1/3 cup of maple syrup in the bowl with beaten eggs. Now mix all the ingredients together. Take the mixture and pour evenly over the cubed bread mixture. Ensure that the bread cubes are nicely dipped in the liquid mixture. Now cover the mixture with an aluminum foil and refrigerate the mixture overnight. Remove the bowl from the refrigerator at least half an hour before baking the next day. Now preheat the oven to 350 degrees F (175 degrees C). Put the baking dish in the oven and bake for 30 minutes. Now remove the aluminum foil from the baking dish and bake for another 30 minutes. Now take a fresh pan and add a cup of sugar, two tablespoons of cornstarch, and one cup of water. Mix the solution and boil while continuously stirring the mixture. Cook for at least 3 minutes. Mix a cup of fresh blueberries to the heated syrup and simmer the haet as the blueberries begin to burst and leave color. Add one tablespoon of butter in the mixture and pour the blueberries sauce over the baked toast. Cut into pieces and serve with maple syrup or the blueberries sauce.

Nutrition:

Proteins: 15.1 g, Carbohydrates: 51.1 g, Fat: 24.8

Plumpy Pumpkin Bread

Preparation Time: 15 minutes | Cooking Time: 1 hour | Servings: 36

Ingredients:

Canned pumpkin puree – 3 cups

Vegetable oil – 1 1/2 cups

Sugar – 4 cups

Eggs – 6

All-purpose flour – 4 3/4 cups

Baking powder – 1 1/2 teaspoons

Baking soda – 1 1/2 teaspoons

Salt – 1 1/2 teaspoons

Cinnamon (ground) – 1 1/2 teaspoons

Nutmeg (ground) – 1 1/2 teaspoons

Cloves (ground) – 1 1/2 teaspoons

Directions:

Start by preheating the oven to 350 degrees F (175 degrees C).

Now take three 9x5 inch loaf pans and grease them using regular cooking spray.

Evenly spray all-purpose flour pan on the greased loaf pans and set them aside.

Now take a fresh large bowl and add 6 eggs into it. Beat them gently into a paste.

Add three cups of canned pumpkin puree, 1 ½ cups of vegetable oil, and four cups of sugar in the bowl with beaten eggs and mix well to form a thick paste.

Now take a big bowl and add 4 3/4 cups of all-purpose flour, 1 ½ teaspoon of baking powder, 1 ½ teaspoon of baking soda, and 1 ½ teaspoon of salt, 1 ½ teaspoon of ground cinnamon, 1 ½ teaspoon of nutmeg, and 1 ½ teaspoon of ground cloves.

Whisk all the ingredients together and add to the pumpkin paste. Stir the mixture until it is evenly blended.

Now place the batter evenly in the greased loaf pans.

Once done, put the greased loaf pans in the preheated oven and bake for at least 50 minutes.

Use a toothpick inserted in the center of the dish to check if it is properly baked or not. Remove the loaf pans from the oven and let it cool for 15-20 minutes. Cut into slices and serve with creamed cheese or nuts of your liking.

Nutrition:

Proteins: 3 g, Carbohydrates: 36.8 g, Fat: 10.3 g

Vintage Pancakes

Preparation Time: 5 minutes | Cooking Time: 15 minutes | Servings: 8

Ingredients:

All-purpose flour – 1 ½ cups

Baking powder – 3 ½ teaspoons

Salt – 1 teaspoon - S ugar – 1 tablespoon

Milk – 1 ¼ cups - Egg – 1

Butter (melted) – 3 tablespoons

Directions:

Begin by taking 1 ½ cups of all-purpose flour in a big fresh bowl. Add 3 ½ teaspoons of baking powder, 1 teaspoon of salt, and 1 teaspoon of sugar into the flour bowl. Now create space in the center of the flour mixture and pour 1 ¼ cups of milk, one egg, and three tablespoons of melted butter. Mix all the ingredients together until you get a smooth batter. Now take a medium frying pan and heat it spraying a little oil over it. Take a quarter cup full f batter and spread over the medium heated frying pan. Spread the batter evenly without leaving any lumps. Heat the cake until the sides start turning golden brown. Flip the pancake using a spatula once you see little bubbles on the surface of the cake. Serve the pancakes hot with a topping of your choice or maple syrup.

Nutrition:

Proteins: 4.5 g, Carbohydrates: 21.7 g, Fat: 5.9 g

Pampered Zucchini Bread

Preparation Time: 20 minutes | Cooking Time: 1 hour | Servings: 24

Ingredients:

All-purpose flour – 3 cups

Salt – 1 teaspoon

Baking soda – 1 teaspoon

Baking powder – 1 teaspoon

Cinnamon (ground) – 3 tablespoon

Eggs – 3

Vegetable oil – 1 cup

Regular sugar – 2 ¼ cups

Vanilla extract – 3 teaspoons

Zucchini (grated) – 2 cups

Walnuts (chopped) – 1 cup

Directions:

Start by preheating the oven to 325 degrees F (165 degrees C).

Now grease a 9 x 4 inch standard baking pans with cooking spray.

Now spray all-purpose flour over the baking pans. Remove any access amount of flour.

Take a fresh medium bowl and add three cups of all-purpose flour, one teaspoon of salt, one teaspoon of baking soda, one teaspoon of baking powder, and three tablespoons of ground cinnamon together.

Now take a fresh big bowl and break three eggs into it.

Add one cup of vegetable oil to the egg bowl along with 2 ¼ cups of regular sugar and a tablespoon of vanilla extract. Beat together all the ingredients in the mixture.

Now empty the all-purpose flour mixture into the beaten egg mixture and stir well to form a thick paste of batter.

Grate three medium-sized zucchini, one cup of chopped walnuts and add to the prepared all-flour batter and stir well.

Now pour the batter evenly into prepared baking pans.

Put the pans in the preheated oven and bake the dish for about 50 minutes.

Use a toothpick to check if the dish is properly baked.

Let the cake cool in the pan for 20 minutes before removing the cake in the pan. Cut into slices of your choice. Leave the remaining cake in the refrigerator.

Nutrition:

Proteins: 3.3 g, Carbohydrates: 32.1 g, Fat: 13.1 g

Lunch Recipes

Shrimp Quesadillas

Preparation Time: 16 minutes | Cooking Time: 5 minutes | Servings: 2

Ingredients:

Two whole wheat tortillas

½ tsp. ground cumin

4 cilantro leaves - 3 oz. diced cooked shrimp

1 de-seeded plump tomato

¾ c. grated non-fat mozzarella cheese

¼ c. diced red onion

Directions:

In medium bowl, combine the grated mozzarella cheese and the warm, cooked shrimp. Add the ground cumin, red onion, and tomato. Mix together. Spread the mixture evenly on the tortillas. Heat a non-stick frying pan. Place the tortillas in the pan, then heat until they crisp. Add the cilantro leaves. Fold over the tortillas. Press down for 1 – 2 minutes. Slice the tortillas into wedges. Serve immediately.

Nutrition:

Calories: 99 Fat: 9 g, Carbs: 7.2 g, Protein: 59 g, Sugars: 4 g, Sodium: 500 mg

The OG Tuna Sandwich

Preparation Time: 15 minutes | Cooking Time: 5 minutes | Servings: 2

Ingredients:

30 g olive oil

1 peeled and diced medium cucumber

2 ½ g pepper

4 whole wheat bread slices

85 g diced onion

2 ½ g salt

1 can flavored tuna   - 85 g shredded spinach

Directions:

Grab your blender and add the spinach, tuna, onion, oil, salt and pepper in, and pulse for about 10 to 20 seconds.   In the meantime, toast your bread and add your diced cucumber to a bowl, which you can pour your tuna mixture in. Carefully mix and add the mixture to the bread once toasted.   Slice in half and serve, while storing the remaining mixture in the fridge.

Nutrition:

Calories: 302 Fat: 5.8 g, Carbs: 36.62 g, Protein: 28 g, Sugars: 3.22 g, Sodium: 445 mg

Easy To Understand Mussels

Preparation Time: 10 minutes | Cooking Time: 10 minutes | Servings: 4

Ingredients:

2 lbs. cleaned mussels

4 minced garlic cloves

2 chopped shallots

Lemon and parsley

2 tbsps. Butter

½ c. broth

½ c. white wine

Directions:

Clean the mussels and remove the beard   Discard any mussels that do not close when tapped against a hard surface   Set your pot to Sauté mode and add chopped onion and butter   Stir and sauté onions   Add garlic and cook for 1 minute   Add broth and wine   Lock up the lid and cook for 5 minutes on HIGH pressure   Release the pressure naturally over 10 minutes   Serve with a sprinkle of parsley and enjoy!

Nutrition:

Calories: 286 Fat: 14 g, Carbs: 12 g Protein: 28 gSugars: 0g Sodium: 314 mg

Chili-Rubbed Tilapia with Asparagus & Lemon

Preparation Time: 10 minutes | Cooking Time: 10 minutes | Servings: 4

Ingredients:

3 tbsps. Lemon juice

2 tbsps. Chili powder

2 tbsps. Extra-virgin olive oil

½ tsp. divided salt

2 lbs. trimmed asparagus

½ tsp. garlic powder

1 lb. tilapia fillets

Directions:

Bring 1 inch of water to a boil in a large saucepan. Put asparagus in a steamer basket, place in the pan, cover and steam until tender-crisp, about 4 minutes.

Transfer to a large plate, spreading out to cool.

Combine chili powder, garlic powder and ¼ teaspoon salt on a plate. Dredge fillets in the spice mixture to coat. Heat oil in a large nonstick skillet over medium-high heat. Add the fish and cook until just opaque in the center, gently turning halfway, and 5 to 7 minutes total.

Divide among 4 plates. Immediately add lemon juice, the remaining ¼ teaspoon salt and asparagus to the pan and cook, stirring constantly, until the asparagus is coated and heated through, about 2 minutes.

Serve the asparagus with the fish.

Nutrition:

Calories: 211, Fat: 10 g, Carbs: 8 g, Protein: 26 g, Sugars: 0.4 g, Sodium: 375.7 mg

Parmesan-Crusted Fish

Preparation Time: 5 minutes | Cooking Time: 7 minutes | Servings: 4

Ingredients:

¾ tsp. ground ginger

1/3 c. panko bread crumbs

Mixed fresh salad greens

¼ c. finely shredded parmesan cheese

1 tbsp. butter

4 skinless cod fillets

3 c. julienned carrots

Directions:

Preheat oven to 450 oF. Lightly coat a baking sheet with nonstick cooking spray.

Rinse and pat dry fish; place on baking sheet. Season with salt and pepper.

In small bowl stir together crumbs and cheese; sprinkle on fish.

Bake, uncovered, 4 to 6 minutes for each 1/2-inch thickness of fish, until crumbs are golden and fish flakes easily when tested with a fork.

Meanwhile, in a large skillet bring 1/2 cup water to boiling; add carrots. Reduce heat.

Cook, covered, for 5 minutes. Uncover; cook 2 minutes more. Add butter and ginger; toss.

Serve fish and carrots with greens.

Nutrition:

Calories: 216.4, Fat: 10.1 g, Carbs: 1.3 g, Protein: 29.0 g, Sugars: 0.1 g, Sodium: 428.3 mg

Lemony Braised Beef Roast

Preparation Time: 15 minutes | Cooking Time: 6-8 hours | Servings: 6

Ingredients:

1 tbsp. minced fresh rosemary

½ c. low-fat, low-sodium beef broth

Freshly ground black pepper

2 lbs. lean beef pot roast

1 sliced onion

2 minced garlic cloves

¼ c. fresh lemon juice

1 tsp. ground cumin

Directions:

In a large slow cooker, add all ingredients and mix well.

Set the slow cooker on low.

Cover and cook for about 6-8 hours.

Nutrition:

Calories: 344 Fat: 2.8 g, Carbs: 18 g, Protein: 32 g, Sugars: 2.4 g, Sodium: 278 mg

Grilled Fennel-cumin Lamb Chops

Preparation Time: 10 minutes | Cooking Time: 15 minutes | Servings: 2

Ingredients:

¼ tsp. salt

1 minced large garlic clove

1/8 tsp. cracked black pepper

¾ tsp. crushed fennel seeds

¼ tsp. ground coriander

4-6 sliced lamb rib chops

¾ tsp. ground cumin

Directions: Trim fat from chops. Place the chops on a plate. In a small bowl combine the garlic, fennel seeds, cumin, salt, coriander, and black pepper. Sprinkle the mixture evenly over chops; rub in with your fingers. Cover the chops with plastic wrap and marinate in the refrigerator at least 30 minutes or up to 24 hours. Grill chops on the rack of an uncovered grill directly over medium coals until chops are desired doneness.

Nutrition:

Calories: 239 Fat: 12 g, Carbs: 2 g Protein: 29 g Sugars: 0 g Sodium: 409 mg

Beef Heart

Preparation Time: 40 minutes | Cooking Time: 30 minutes | Servings: 4

Ingredients:

1 chopped large onion

1 c. water

2 peeled and chopped tomatoes

1 boiled beef heart

2 tbsps. tomato paste

Directions:

Boil the beef heart until half-done.

Sauté the onions with tomatoes until soft.

Cut the beef heart into cubes and add to tomato and onion mixture. Add water and tomato paste. Stew on low heat for 30 minutes.

Nutrition:

Calories: 138 Fat: 3 g Carbs: 0.1 g, Protein: 24.2 g, Sugars: 0 g, Sodium: 50.2 mg

Jerk Beef and Plantain Kabobs

Preparation Time: 10 minutes | Cooking Time: 15 minutes | Servings: 4

Ingredients:

2 peeled and sliced ripe plantains

2 tbsps. Red wine vinegar

Lime wedges

1 tbsp. cooking oil - 1 sliced medium red onion

12 oz. sliced boneless beef sirloin steak

1 tbsp. Jamaican jerk seasoning

Directions:

Trim fat from meat. Cut into 1-inch pieces. In a small bowl, stir together red wine vinegar, oil, and jerk seasoning. Toss meat cubes with half of the vinegar mixture. On long skewers, alternately thread meat, plantain chunks, and onion wedges, leaving a 1/4-inch space between pieces. Brush plantains and onion wedges with remaining vinegar mixture. Place skewers on the rack of an uncovered grill directly over medium coals. Grill for 12 to 15 minutes or until meat is desired doneness, turning occasionally. Serve with lime wedges.

Nutrition:

Calories: 260 Fat: 7 g, Carbs: 21 g Protein: 26 g Sugars: 2.5 g Sodium: 358 mg

Beef Pot

Preparation Time: 10 minutes | Cooking Time: 40 minutes | Servings: 2

Ingredients:

4 tbsps. Sour cream

¼ shredded cabbage head

1 tsp. butter

2 peeled and sliced carrots

1 chopped onion

10 oz. boiled and sliced beef tenderloin

1 tbsp. flour

Directions:

Sauté the cabbage, carrots and onions in butter.

Spray a pot with cooking spray.

In layers place the sautéed vegetables, then beef, then another layer of vegetables. Beat the sour cream with flour until smooth and pour over the beef. Cover and bake at 400F for 40 minutes.

Nutrition:

Calories: 210 Fat: 30 g, Carbs: 4 g Protein: 14 g Sugars: 1 g Sodium: 600 mg

Cheesy Black Bean Wraps

Preparation Time: 10 minutes | Cooking Time: 5 minutes | Servings: 6

Ingredients:

2 Tablespoons Green Chili Peppers, Chopped

4 Green Onions, Diced

1 Tomato, Diced

1 Tablespoon Garlic, Chopped

6 Tortilla Wraps, Whole Grain & Fat Free

¾ Cup Cheddar Cheese, Shredded

¾ Cup Salsa

1 ½ Cups Corn Kernels

3 Tablespoons Cilantro, Fresh & Chopped

1 ½ Cup Black Beans, Canned & Drained

Directions:

Toss your chili peppers, corn, black beans, garlic, tomato, onions and cilantro in a bowl.

Heat the mixture in a microwave for a minute, and stir for a half a minute.

Spread the two tortillas between paper towels and microwave for twenty seconds. Warm the remaining tortillas the same way, and add a half a cup of bean mixture, two tablespoons of salsa and two tablespoons of cheese for each tortilla. Roll them up before serving.

Nutrition:

Calories: 341, Protein: 19 Grams, Fat: 11 Grams, Carbs: 36.5 Grams, Sodium: 141 mg, Cholesterol: 0 mg

Arugula Risotto

Preparation Time: 10 minutes | Cooking Time: 15 minutes | Servings: 4

Ingredients:

1 Tablespoon Olive Oil

½ Cup Yellow Onion, Chopped

1 Cup Quinoa, Rinsed

1 Clove Garlic, Minced

2 ½ Cups Vegetable Stock, Low Sodium

2 Cups Arugula, Chopped & Stemmed

1 Carrot, Peeled & shredded

½ Cup Shiitake Mushrooms, Sliced

¼ Teaspoon Black Pepper

¼ Teaspoon Sea Salt, Fine

¼ Cup Parmesan Cheese, Grated

Directions:

Get a saucepan and place it over medium heat, heating up your oil. Cook for four minutes until your onions are softened, and then add in your garlic and quinoa. Cook for a minute.

Stir in your stock, and bring it to a boil. Reduce it to simmer, and cook for twelve minutes.

Add in your arugula, mushrooms and carrots, cooking for an additional two minutes.

Add in salt, pepper and cheese before serving.

Nutrition:

Calories: 288, Protein: 6 Grams, Fat: 5 Grams, Carbs: 28 Grams, Sodium: 739 mg, Cholesterol: 0.5 mg

Vegetarian Stuffed Eggplant

Preparation Time: 20 minutes | Cooking Time: 15 minutes | Servings: 2

Ingredients:

4 Ounces White Beans, Cooked

1 Tablespoons Olive Oil

1 cup Water

1 Eggplant

¼ Cup Onion, Chopped

½ Cup Bell Pepper, Chopped

1 Cup Canned Tomatoes, Unsalted

¼ Cup Tomato Liquid

¼ Cup Celery, Chopped

1 Cup Mushrooms, Fresh & Sliced

¾ Cup Breadcrumbs, Whole Wheat

Black Pepper to Taste

Directions:

Preheat the oven to 350, and then grease a baking dish with cooking spray.

Trim the eggplant and cut it in half lengthwise. Scoop the pulp out using a spoon, leaving a shell that's a quarter of an inch thick.

Place the shells in the baking dish with their cut side up.

Add the water to the bottom of the dish, and dice the eggplant pulp into cubes, setting them to the side.

Add the oil into an iron skillet, heating it over medium heat.

Stir in peppers, chopped eggplants, and onions with your celery, mushrooms, tomatoes and tomato juice.

Cook for ten minutes on simmering heat, and then stir in your bread crumbs, beans and black pepper. Divide the mixture between eggshells.

Cover with foil, and bake for fifteen minutes. Serve warm.

Nutrition:

Calories: 334, Protein: 26 Grams, Fat: 10 Grams, Carbs: 35 Grams, Sodium: 142 mg, Cholesterol: 162 mg

Vegetable Tacos

Preparation Time: 15 minutes | Cooking Time: 15 minutes | Servings: 4

Ingredients:

1 Tablespoon Olive Oil

1 Cup Red Onion, Chopped

1 Cup Yellow Summer Squash, Diced

1 Cup Green Zucchini, Diced

3 Cloves Garlic, Minced

4 Tomatoes, Seeded& Chopped

1 Jalapeno Chili, Seeded & Chopped

1 Cup Corn Kernels, Fresh

1 Cup Pinto Beans, Canned, Rinsed & Drained

½ Cup Cilantro, Fresh & Chopped

8 Corn Tortillas

½ Cup Smoke Flavored Salsa

Directions:

Get out a saucepan and add in your olive oil over medium heat, and stir in your onion. Cook until softened.

Add in your squash and zucchini, cooking for an additional five minutes.

Stir in your garlic, beans, tomatoes, jalapeño and corn. Cook for an additional five minutes before stirring in your cilantro and removing the pan from heat.

Warm each tortilla, in a nonstick skillet for twenty seconds per side.

Place the tortillas on a serving plate, spooning the vegetable mixture into each. Top with salsa, and roll to serve.

Nutrition:

Calories: 310, Protein: 10 Grams, Fat: 6 Grams, Carbs: 54 Grams, Sodium: 97 mg, Cholesterol: 20 mg

Fruit Chicken Salad

Preparation Time: 45 minutes | Cooking Time: 45 minutes | Servings: 8

Ingredients:

Boneless chicken breast halves – 4 skinless

Diced stalk celery – 1 cup

Green onions – 4

Golden apple – 1

Golden raisins – 1/3 cup

Seedless green grapes – 1/3 cup

Chopped toasted pecans – 1/2 cup

Ground black pepper – 1/8 teaspoon

Curry powder – 1/2 teaspoon

Light mayonnaise – 3/4 cup

Directions:

Start by taking four boneless chicken breast halves and cut them into equal tiny cubes.

Now take a pan and cook chicken cubes well. Do not overcook.

Take four green onions and chop them into pieces.

One cup of thin-sliced diced stalk celery, four chopped green onions, one peeled golden apple, 1/3 cup of golden raisins, 1/3 cup of seedless green grapes chopped in two halves, 1/2 cup of chopped toasted pecans, 1/8 teaspoon of ground black pepper, 1/2 teaspoon of Curry powder

Now lightly mix all ingredients put into the bowl. Avoid mashing.

Keep the bowl aside for at least two minutes.

Now add 3/4 cup of light mayonnaise in the bowl and gently mix the mixture. Ensure that the spread is evenly divided

Cover the bowl with plastic film and put it in the refrigerator for half an hour.

Serve before it gets soggy.

The salad tastes well when kept overnight.

Nutrition:

Calories: 229, Proteins: 15.1 g, Carbohydrates: 12.3 g, Fat: 14 g

Whole Grain Pasta with Meat Sauce

Preparation Time: 10 minutes | Cooking Time: 30 minutes | Servings: 6

Ingredients:

Whole-grain pasta – 1 pound

Extra-lean ground beef – 1 pound

Onion – 1, diced

Garlic – 3 cloves, minced

No-salt-added tomato sauce – 2 (8-ounce) cans

Red wine – 1/3 cup

Balsamic vinegar – 1 Tbsp.

Dried basil - 1 tsp.

Dried marjoram – ½ tsp.

Dried oregano – ½ tsp.

Dried red pepper flakes - ½ tsp.

Dried thyme - ½ tsp.

Freshly ground black pepper - ½ tsp.

Directions:

Follow the direction on the package and cook the pasta. Omit the salt. Drain and set aside.

Place onion, ground beef and garlic in a pan over medium heat. Stir-fry for 5 minutes, or until the beef has browned.

Add remaining ingredients and stir to combine. Simmer, uncovered, for 10 minutes, stirring occasionally.

Remove from heat and spoon over pasta.

Serve.

Nutrition:

Calories: 387, Fat: 5g, Carb: 58g, Protein: 27g, Sodium 65mg

Beef Tacos

Preparation Time: 10 minutes | Cooking Time: 20 minutes | Servings: 6

Ingredients:

Extra-lean ground beef – 1 pound

Large onion – 1, chopped

Garlic – 2 cloves, minced

No-salt-added tomato sauce – 1 (8-ounce) can

Low-sodium Worcestershire sauce – 2 tsp.

Molasses - 1 Tbsp.

Apple cider vinegar – 1 Tbsp.

Ground cumin – 1 Tbsp.

Ground sweet paprika – 1 Tbsp.

Dried red pepper flakes - ½ tsp.

Ground black pepper to taste

Low-sodium taco shells – 1 package

Chopped fresh cilantro - ¼ cup

Tomato and lettuce of serving

Directions:

Place the ground beef, onion, and garlic in a pan over medium heat.

Stir-fry for 5 minutes or until the beef is browned.

Lower heat to medium-low and add the Worcestershire sauce, tomato sauce, molasses, vinegar, cumin, red pepper flakes, paprika, and black pepper. Simmer, stirring frequently, about 10 minutes.

Heat taco shells according to package directions. Set aside.

Remove the sauté pan from the heat. Stir in cilantro.

Divide evenly between the taco shells.

Garnish with lettuce, tomato and serve.

Nutrition:

Calories: 255, Fat: 9g, Carb: 23g, Protein: *18*g, Sodium 79mg

Dirty Rice

Preparation Time: 10 minutes | Cooking Time: 30 minutes | Servings: 4

Ingredients:

Extra-lean ground beef - ½ pound

Large onion – 1, diced

Celery – 2 stalks, diced

Garlic – 2 cloves, minced

Bell pepper – 1, diced

Sodium-free beef bouillon granules - 1 tsp.

Water - 1 cup

Low-sodium Worcestershire sauce – 2 tsp.

Dried thyme – 1 ½ tsp.

Dried basil – 1 tsp.

Dried marjoram - ½ tsp.

Ground black pepper - ¼ tsp.

Pinch ground cayenne pepper

Scallions – 2, diced

Cooked long-grain brown rice – 3 cups

Directions:

In a pan, place the onion, ground beef, celery, and garlic. Stir-fry for 5 minutes or until beef is browned.

Add beef bouillon, bell pepper, water, sauce, and herbs and stir to combine.

Bring to a boil.

Then reduce heat to low, and cover.

Simmer for 20 minutes.

Stir in the scallions and simmer, uncovered, for 3 minutes.

Remove from heat. Add cooked rice and stir to combine.

Serve.

Nutrition:

Calories: 272, Fat: 4g, Carb: 41g, Protein: 16g, Sodium 92mg

Beef with Pea Pods

Preparation Time: 5 minutes | Cooking Time: 10 minutes | Servings: 4

Ingredients:

Thin beef steak – ¾ pound, sliced into thin strips

Peanut oil – 1 Tbsp.

Scallions – 3, sliced

Garlic – 2 cloves, minced

Minced fresh ginger – 2 tsp.

Fresh pea pods – 4 cups, trimmed

Homemade soy sauce – 3 Tbsp.

Cooked brown rice – 4 cups

Directions:

Heat the oil in a pan. Add the garlic, scallions, and ginger. Stir-fry for 30 seconds. Add the sliced beef and stir-fry for 5 minutes, or until beef has browned. Add pea pods and soy sauce and stir-fry for 3 minutes. Remove from heat. Serve with rice.

Nutrition:

Calories: 466 Fat: 11g Carb: 64g Protein: 27g Sodium 71mg

Whole-Grain Rotini with Ground Pork

Preparation Time: 10 minutes | Cooking Time: 25 minutes | Servings: 6

Ingredients:

Whole-grain rotini - 1 (13-ounce) package

Lean ground pork – 1 pound

Red onion – 1, chopped

Garlic – 3 cloves, minced

Bell pepper – 1, chopped

Pumpkin puree – 1 cup

Ground sage – 2 tsp.

Ground rosemary – 1 tsp.

Ground black pepper to taste

Directions:

Cook the pasta (follow the package insturctions). Omit salt, drain and set aside.Heat a pan over medium heat. Add onion, garlic, and ground pork and sauté for 2 minutes.Add bell pepper and sauté for 5 minutes. Remove from heat. Add pasta to the pan along with remaining ingredients. Mix and serve.

Nutrition:

Calories: 331 Fat: 7g Carb: 45g Protein: 23g Sodium 48mg

Roasted Pork Loin with Herbs

Preparation Time: 20 minutes | Cooking Time: 1 hour | Servings: 4

Ingredients:

Boneless pork loin roast – 2 lbs.

Garlic – 3 cloves, minced

Dried rosemary – 1 Tbsp.

Dried thyme – 1 tsp.

Dried basil – 1 tsp.

Salt – ¼ tsp.

Olive oil – ¼ cup

White wine – ½ cup

Pepper to taste

Directions:

Preheat the oven to 350F.

Crush the garlic with thyme, rosemary, basil, salt, and pepper, making a paste. Set aside.

Use a knife to pierce meat several times.

Press the garlic paste into the slits.

Rub the meat with the rest of the garlic mixture and olive oil.

Place pork loin into the oven, turning and basting with pan liquids, until the pork reaches 145F, about 1 hour. Remove the pork from the oven.

Place the pan over heat and add white wine, stirring the brown bits on the bottom.

Top roast with sauce.

Serve.

Nutrition:

Calories: 464, Fat: 20.7g, Carb: 2.4g, Protein: 59.6g, Sodium 279mg

Garlic Lime Pork Chops

Preparation Time: 20 minutes | Cooking Time: 10 minutes | Servings: 4

Ingredients:

Lean boneless pork chops – 4 (6-oz. each)

Garlic – 4 cloves, crushed

Cumin – ½ tsp.

Chili powder - ½ tsp.

Paprika - ½ tsp.

Juice of ½ lime

Lime zest – 1 tsp.

Kosher salt - ¼ tsp.

Fresh pepper to taste

Directions:

In a bowl, season pork with cumin, chili powder, paprika, garlic salt, and pepper. Add lime juice and zest. Marinate the pork for 20 minutes. Line a broiler pan with foil. Place the pork chops on the broiler pan and broil for 5 minutes on each side or until browned. Serve.

Nutrition:

Calories: 233 Fat: 13.2g Carb: 4.3g Protein: 25.5g Sodium 592mg

Lamb Curry with Tomatoes and Spinach

Preparation Time: 10 minutes | Cooking Time: 12 minutes | Servings: 4

Ingredients:

Olive oil – 1 tsp.

Lean boneless lamb – 1 pound, sliced thinly

Onion – 1, chopped

Garlic – 3 cloves, minced

Red bell pepper – 1, chopped

Salt-free tomato paste – 2 Tbsp.

Salt-free curry powder – 1 Tbsp.

No-salt-added diced tomatoes – 1(15-ounce) can

Fresh baby spinach – 10 ounces

Low-sodium beef or vegetable broth - ½ cup

Red wine – ¼ cup

Chopped fresh cilantro – ¼ cup

Ground black pepper to taste

Directions:

Heat the oil in a pan.

Add lamb and brown both sides, about 2 minutes.

Add garlic, onion, and bell pepper. Stir-fry for 2 minutes. Stir in the curry powder and tomato paste.

Add the tomatoes with juice, spinach, broth, and wine and stir to mix.

Stir-fry for 3 to 4 minutes and lamb has cooked through.

Remove from heat. Season with pepper and stir in cilantro.

Serve.

Nutrition:

Calories: 238, Fat: 7g, Carb: 14g, Protein: 27g, Sodium 167mg

Pomegranate-Marinated Leg of Lamb

Preparation Time: 10 minutes | Cooking Time: 20 minutes | Servings: 6

Ingredients:

Bottled pomegranate juice - ½ cup

Hearty red wine – ½ cup

Ground cumin - 1 tsp.

Dried oregano – 1 tsp.

Crushed hot red pepper – ½ tsp.

Garlic – 3 cloves, minced

For the lamb

Boneless leg of lamb – 1 ¾ pound, butterflied and fat trimmed

Kosher salt – ½ tsp.

Olive oil spray

Directions:

To make the marinade, whisk everything in a bowl and transfer to a zippered plastic bag.

To prepare the lamb: add the lamb to the bag, press out the air, and close the bag. Marinate for 1 hour in the refrigerator.

Preheat the broiler (8 inches from the source of heat).

Remove the lamb from the marinade, blot with paper towels, but do not dry completely.

Season with salt. Spray the broiler rack with oil.

Place the lamb on the rack and broil, turning occasionally, about 20 minutes, or until lamb is browned and reaches 130F.

Remove from heat, slice and serve with carving juices on top.

Nutrition:

Calories: 273, Fat: 15g, Carb: 0g, Protein: 31g, Sodium 219mg

Beef Fajitas with Peppers

Preparation Time: 10 minutes | Cooking Time: 12 minutes | Servings: 6

Ingredients:

Olive oil – 2 tsp. plus more for the spray

Sirloin steak – 1 pound, cut into bite-size pieces

Red bell pepper – 1, chopped

Green bell pepper – 1, chopped

Red onion – 1, chopped

Garlic - 2 cloves, minced

DASH friendly Mexican seasoning – 1 Tbsp. (or any seasoning without salt)

Boston lettuce leaves – 12 for serving

Lime wedges or corn tortillas for serving

Directions:

Heat oil in a skillet.

Add half of the sirloin and cook until browned on both sides, about 2 minutes. Transfer to a plate.

Then repeat with the remaining sirloin.

Heat the 2 tsp. oil in the skillet.

Add onion, bell peppers, and garlic, cook and stir for 7 minutes or until tender.

Stir in the beef with any juices and the seasoning. Transfer to a plate.

Fill lettuce lead with beef mixture and drizzle lime juice on top.

Roll up and serve.

Nutrition:

Calories: 231, Fat: 12g, Carb: 6g, Protein: 24g, Sodium 59mg

Dinner Recipes

Pork Medallions with Herbs de Provence

Preparation Time: 5 minutes | Cooking Time: 10 minutes | Servings: 2

Ingredients:

Pork tenderloin – 8 ounces, cut into 6 pieces (crosswise)

Ground black pepper to taste

Herbs de Provence – ½ tsp.

Dry white wine – ¼ cup

Directions:

Season the pork with black pepper.

Place the pork between waxed paper sheets and roll with a rolling pin until about ¼ inch thick.

Cook the pork in a pan for 2 to 3 minutes on each side.

Remove from heat and season with the herb. Place the pork on plates and keep warm. Cook the wine in the pan until boiling. Scrape to get the brown bits from the bottom. Serve pork with the sauce.

Nutrition:

Calories: 120 Fat: 2g Carb: 1g Protein: 24g Sodium 62mg

Baked Chicken

Preparation Time: 10 minutes | Cooking Time: 1 hour | Servings: 4

Ingredients:

Chicken – 3 to 4 pound, cut into parts

Olive oil – 3 Tbsp.

Thyme – ½ tsp.

Sea salt – ¼ tsp.

Ground black pepper

Low-sodium chicken stock – ½ cup

Directions:

Preheat the oven to 400F.

Rub oil over chicken pieces. Sprinkle with salt, thyme, and pepper.

Place chicken in the roasting pan.

Bake in the oven for 30 minutes.

Then lower the heat to 350F.

Bake for 15 to 30 minutes more or until juice runs clear. Serve.

Nutrition:

Calories: 550 Fat: 19g Carb: 0g Protein: 91g Sodium 480mg

Orange Chicken and Broccoli Stir-Fry

Preparation Time: 10 minutes | Cooking Time: 15 minutes | Servings: 4

Ingredients:

Olive oil – 1 Tbsp.

Chicken breast – 1 pound, boneless and skinless, cut into strips

Orange juice – 1/3 cup

Homemade soy sauce - 2 Tbsp.

Cornstarch – 2 tsp.

Broccoli – 2 cups, cut into small pieces

Snow peas – 1 cup - Cabbage – 2 cups, shredded

Brown rice – 2 cups, cooked - Sesame seeds – 1 Tbsp.

Directions: Combine the orange juice, soy sauce, and corn starch in a bowl. Set aside. Heat oil in a pan. Add chicken.Stir-fry until the chicken is golden brown on all sides, about 5 minutes. Add snow peas, cabbage, broccoli, and sauce mixture. Continue to stir-fry for 8 minutes or until vegetables are tender but still crisp.

Nutrition:

Calories: 340 Fat: 8g Carb: 35g Protein: 28g Sodium 240mg

Mediterranean Lemon Chicken and Potatoes

Preparation Time: 10 minutes | Cooking Time: 30 minutes | Servings: 4

Ingredients:

Chicken breast – 1 ½ pound, skinless and boneless, cut into 1-inch cubes

Yukon Gold potatoes – 1 pound, cut into cubes

Onion – 1, chopped

Red pepper – 1, chopped

Low-sodium vinaigrette – ½ cup

Lemon juice – ¼ cup

Oregano – 1 tsp.

Garlic powder – ½ tsp.

Chopped tomato – ½ cup

Ground black pepper to taste

Directions:

Preheat oven to 400F.

Except for the tomatoes, mix everything in a bowl.

On 4 aluminum foils, place an equal amount of chicken and potato mixture. Fold to make packets.

Bake at 400F for 30 minutes. Open packets.

Top with chopped tomatoes.

Season with black pepper to taste.

Nutrition:

Calories: 320, Fat: 4g, Carb: 34g, Protein: 43g, Sodium 420mg

Tandoori Chicken

Preparation Time: 10 minutes | Cooking Time: 20 minutes | Servings: 6

Ingredients:

Nonfat yogurt – 1 cup, plain

Lemon juice – ½ cup

Garlic – 5 cloves, crushed

Paprika – 2 Tbsp.

Curry powder – 1 tsp.

Ground ginger – 1 tsp.

Red pepper flakes – 1 tsp.

Chicken breasts – 6, skinless and boneless, cut into 2-inch chunks

Wooden skewers – 6, soaked in water

Directions:

Preheat the oven to 400F.

In a bowl, combine lemon juice, yogurt, garlic, and spices. Blend well.

Divide chicken and thread onto skewers. Place skewers in a baking dish.

Pour half of the yogurt mixture onto chicken. Cover and marinate in the refrigerator for 20 minutes

Spray a baking dish with cooking spray.

Place chicken skewers in the pan and coat with the remaining ½ of yogurt marinade.

Bake in the oven until chicken is cooked, about 15 to 20 minutes.

Serve with veggies or brown rice.

Nutrition:

Calories: 175, Fat: 2g, Carb: 8g, Protein: 30g, Sodium 105mg

Mighty Garlic and Butter Sword Fish

Preparation Time: 10 minutes | Cooking Time: 2 hours and 30 minutes | Servings: 4

Ingredients:

½ c. melted butter

6 chopped garlic cloves

1 tbsp. black pepper

5 sword fish fillets

Directions:

Take a mixing bowl and toss in all of your garlic, black pepper alongside the melted butter

Take a parchment paper and place your fish fillet in that paper

Cover it up with the butter mixture and wrap up the fish

Repeat the process until all of your fish are wrapped up

Let it cook for 2 and a half hours and release the pressure naturally

Serve

Nutrition:

Calories: 379, Fat: 26 g Carbs: 1 g Protein: 34 g Sugars: 0 g Sodium: 666 mg

Supreme Cooked Lobster

Preparation Time: 10 minutes | Cooking Time: 7 minutes | Servings: 4

Ingredients:

1 c. white wine

1 c. water

2 lobster pieces

Directions:

Add the listed ingredients to your Instant Pot

Lock up the lid and cook on HIGH pressure for 7 minutes

Release the pressure naturally

Open and add some extra melted butter

Serve and enjoy!

Nutrition:

Calories: 231, Fat: 9 g, Carbs: 5 g, Protein: 30 g, Sugars: 0 g, Sodium: 551 mg

Tilapia with Parsley

Preparation Time: 10 minutes | Cooking Time: 1 hour and 30 minutes | Servings: 6

Ingredients:

2 tbsps. Melted low-fat unsalted butter

1 tsp. garlic powder

¼ c. chopped fresh parsley

Freshly ground black pepper

4 oz. tilapia fillets

3 tsps. Grated fresh lemon rind

Directions:

Grease a slow cooker.

Sprinkle the tilapia fillets with garlic powder and black pepper generously.

Place lemon rind and parsley over fillets evenly.

Drizzle with melted butter. Set the slow cooker on low. Cover and cook for about 1½ hours.

Nutrition:

Calories: 239.1 Fat: 4.3 g, Carbs: 22.3 g, Protein: 33.7 g, Sugars: 0 g Sodium: 381 mg

Thai Coconut Tilapia and Rice

Preparation Time: 15 minutes | Cooking Time: 25 minutes | Servings: 4

Ingredients:

170 g chopped baby spinach

425 g coconut milk

2 ½ g salted butter

680 g jasmine

2 ½ g chili flakes

4 coconut crusted tilapia fillets

680 g coconut water

Directions:

Preheat the oven to 400 ₀F and place fish in a lightly greased pan. Bake for 25 minutes.

In the meantime, put your rice in a pot to cook with coconut water, coconut milk, and a dash of salt. Set the pot at medium heat for about 2 minutes, till it reaches boiling point, then put the heat down and let the rice simmer for about twenty more minutes.

Add the chili flakes in now, to allow the rice to fully take in the flavor. Just before you are ready to serve, add in the spinach and stir for about 3 to 4 minutes, before straining both, and plating.

Take the fish out of the oven, slice, and serve over the coconut rice.

Nutrition:

Calories: 190, Fat: 3.4 g, Carbs: 35.67 g, Protein: 6 g, Sugars: 1.7 g, Sodium: 256.2 mg

Nutmeg Pork Chops

Preparation Time: 10 minutes | Cooking Time: 35 minutes | Servings: 3

Ingredients:

1 chopped yellow onion

1 tbsp. balsamic vinegar

½ c. organic olive oil

3 boneless pork chops

8 oz. sliced mushrooms

2 tsps. Ground nutmeg

¼ c. coconut milk

1 tsp. garlic powder

Directions: Heat up a pan using the oil over medium heat, add mushrooms and onions, stir and cook for 5 minutes.   Add pork chops, nutmeg and garlic powder and cook for 5 minutes more.   Add vinegar and coconut milk, toss, introduce inside oven and bake at 350 ₀F and bake for a half-hour.   Divide between plates and serve.   Enjoy!

Nutrition:

Calories: 260, Fat: 10 g, Carbs: 8 g, Protein: 22 g, Sugars: 2.4 , Sodium: 78 mg

Butter and Dill Pork Chops

Preparation Time: 5 minutes | Cooking Time: 26 minutes | Servings: 4

Ingredients:

½ c. chicken broth

½ c. white wine

4 bone-in pork loin pieces

2 tbsps. unflavored vinegared butter

1 tbsp. minced fresh dill fronds

½ tsp. flavored vinegar

½ tsp. ground black pepper

16 baby carrots

Directions:

The first step here is to set your pot to sauté mode

Season the chops with pepper and flavored vinegar

Toss your chops into your pot and cook for 4 minutes

Transfer the chops to a plate and repeat to cook and brown the rest

Pour in 1 tablespoon of butter and Toss in your carrots, dill to the cooker and let it cook for about 1 minute

Pour in the wine and scrape off any browned bits in your cooker while the liquid comes to a boil

Stir in the broth

Return the chops to your pot

Lock up the lid and let it cook for about 18 minutes at high pressure

Naturally release the pressure by keeping it aside for 8 minutes

Unlock and serve with some sauce poured over

Nutrition:

Calories: 296, Fat: 25 g, Carbs: 0 g, Protein: 17 g, Sugars: 1.3 g, Sodium: 155 mg

Paprika Pork with Carrots

Preparation Time: 10 minutes | Cooking Time: 30 minutes | Servings: 4

Ingredients:

1 sliced red onion

1 lb. cubed pork stew meat

2 tbsps. olive oil

¼ c. low-sodium veggie stock

Black pepper

2 peeled and sliced carrots

2 tsps. sweet paprika

Directions:

Heat up a pan with the oil over medium heat, add the onion, stir and sauté for 5 minutes.

Add the meat, toss and brown for 5 minutes more.

Add the rest of the ingredients, bring to a simmer and cook over medium heat for 20 minutes. Divide the mix between plates and serve.

Nutrition:

Calories: 328, Fat: 18.1 g Carbs: 6.4 g Protein: 34 g Sugars: 14 g Sodium: 399 mg

Pork and Greens Mix

Preparation Time: 10 minutes | Cooking Time: 20 minutes | Servings: 4

Ingredients:

4 oz. mixed salad greens

1 tbsp. chopped chives

1/3 c. coconut aminos

2 tbsps. balsamic vinegar

1 tbsp. olive oil

4 oz. sliced pork stew meat

1 c. halved cherry tomatoes

Directions:

Heat up a pan with the oil over medium heat, add the pork, aminos and the vinegar, toss and cook for 15 minutes.

Add the salad greens and the other ingredients, toss, cook for 5 minutes more, divide between plates and serve.

Nutrition:

Calories: 125 Fat: 6.4 g, Carbs: 6.8 g Protein: 9.1 g Sugars: 0.2 g Sodium: 388.6 mg

Sage Pork Chops

Preparation Time: 10 minutes | Cooking Time: 35 minutes | Servings: 4

Ingredients:

2 tbsps. olive oil

1 tbsp. lemon juice

4 pork chops

1 tbsp. chopped sage

Black pepper

1 tsp. smoked paprika

2 minced garlic cloves

Directions:

In a baking dish, combine the pork chops with the oil and the other ingredients, toss, introduce in the oven and bake at 400 oF for 35 minutes.

Divide the pork chops between plates and serve with a side salad.

Nutrition:

Calories: 263, Fat: 12.4 g Carbs: 22.2 g Protein: 16 g Sugars: 0 g Sodium: 960 mg

Pork with Avocados

Preparation Time: 10 minutes | Cooking Time: 15 minutes | Servings: 4

Ingredients:

1 c. halved cherry tomatoes

½ c. low-sodium veggie stock

1 tbsp. olive oil

2 c. baby spinach

1 lb. sliced pork steak

2 peeled, pitted and sliced avocados

1 tbsp. balsamic vinegar

Directions:

Heat up a pan with the oil over medium-high heat, add the meat, toss and cook for 10 minutes.

Add the spinach and the other ingredients, toss, cook for 5 minutes more, divide into bowls and serve.

Nutrition:

Calories: 390, Fat: 12.5 g Carbs: 16.8 g Protein: 13.5 g Sugars: 1 g Sodium: 0 mg

Simple Roast

Preparation Time: 10 minutes | Cooking Time: 45 minutes | Servings: 6

Ingredients:

3 Cloves Garlic, Minced

Black Pepper to Taste

1 Cup Beef Stock, Low Sodium

2 Yellow Onions, Chopped Roughly

4 lbs. Chuck Roast, Lean & Fat Removed

1 Thyme Sprig, Fresh & Chopped

2 Carrots, Sliced

3 Bay Leaves

2 Celery Stalks, Chopped

Directions:

Mix everything in your instant pot and then seal the lid. Cook on high pressure for forty-five minutes, and then slice the roast to serve.

Nutrition:

Calories: 351 Protein: 14 Grams Fat: 7 Grams Carbs: 20 Grams

Easy Chili

Preparation Time: 10 minutes | Cooking Time: 15 minutes | Servings: 4

Ingredients:

1 Tablespoon Chili Powder

1 Tablespoon Cumin

1 lb. Chicken, Ground

2 Cloves Garlic, Minced

1 Tablespoon Avocado Oil

1 Yellow Onion, Chopped

1 Teaspoon Cocoa Powder

2 Tablespoons Tomato Paste

1 Cup Chicken Stock, Low Sodium

1 Teaspoon Oregano

2 Cups Corn

Black Pepper to Taste

28 Ounces Tomatoes, Canned & No Salt

28 Ounces Kidney Beans, Canned, No Salt, Drained & Rinsed

Directions:

Mix everything together in your instant pot and then stir well. Seal the lid, and cook on high pressure for fifteen minutes.

Finish with a quick release and then serve warm.

Nutrition:

Calories: 265, Protein: 7 Grams, Fat: 6 Grams, Carbs: 19 Grams

Italian Shrimp Dinner

Preparation Time: 15 minutes | Cooking Time: 15 minutes | Servings: 4

Ingredients:

8 Ounces Mushrooms, Chopped

1 lb. Shrimp, Peeled & Deveined

1 Yellow Onion, Chopped

1 Asparagus Bunch, Chopped

Black Pepper to Taste

2 Tablespoons Olive Oil

2 Teaspoons Italian Seasoning

1 Teaspoon Red Pepper Flakes, Crushed

1 Cup Cheddar Cheese, Fat Free & Grated

2 Cloves Garlic, Minced

1 Cup Coconut Cream

1 Cup Water

Directions:

Add the steamer basket to your instant pot after filling with one cup water.

Add the asparagus in the basket, and seal the lid. Cook on high pressure for three minutes, and then use a quick release. Submerge it in ice water to stop the asparagus from cooking, and drain before setting it aside.

Clean the instant pot and then press sauté. Add oil, and once it' shot cook your onion and mushrooms for four minutes. Add pepper flakes, Italian seasoning and the asparagus back in. stir well, and cook for a few minutes.

Add the cheddar, garlic, shrimp and coconut cream. Cover and cook on high pressure for four minutes. Serve warm.

Nutrition:

Calories: 275, Protein: 8 Grams, Fat: 6 Grams, Carbs: 17 Grams

Cabbage & Beef Stew

Preparation Time: 1 hour and 14 minutes | Cooking Time: 16 minutes | Servings: 6

Ingredients:

4 Carrots, Chopped

4 Cups Water

1 Cabbage Head, Shredded

3 Cloves Garlic, Chopped

Black Pepper to Taste

2 Bay Leaves

2 ½ lbs. Beef Brisket, Fat Removed

Directions:

Place your brisket in the instant pot with water, pepper, bay leaves and garlic. Seal the lid and cook on high pressure for one hour.

Use a quick release, and then add the cabbage, carrot, and stir well. Cook on high pressure for six minutes, and then use a natural pressure release for ten minutes. Follow with a quick release and serve warm.

Nutrition:

Calories: 281 Protein: 8, Grams Fat: 8 Grams, Carbs: 21 Grams

Fish Curry

Preparation Time: 10 minutes | Cooking Time: 10 minutes | Servings: 6

Ingredients:

2 Onions, Sliced

2 Cloves Garlic, Minced

6 Curry Leaves

14 Ounces Coconut Milk

1 Tomato, Chopped

1 Tablespoon Olive Oil

6 White Fish Fillets, Skinless, Boneless & Chopped

1 Tablespoon Coriander, Ground

1 Tablespoon Ginger, Grated

½ Teaspoon Turmeric

Black Pepper to taste

2 Tablespoons Lemon Juice, Fresh

½ Teaspoon Fenugreek, Ground

Directions:

Press sauté and add the curry leaves and oil. Fry for a minute before adding the garlic, coriander, onion, ginger, turmeric, coconut milk, tomatoes, fish and fenugreek. Stir well, and then seal the lid.

Cook on low pressure for ten minutes before using a quick release.

Add the black pepper and stir well. Serve drizzled with lemon juice.

Nutrition:

Calories: 281, Protein: 7 Grams, Fat: 6 Grams, Carbs: 14 Grams

Beef Bourguignon

Preparation Time: 10 minutes | Cooking Time: 30 minutes | Servings: 4

Ingredients:

1 lb. Stewing Steak

½ lb. Bacon

5 Carrots

1 Red Onion, Sliced

2 Cloves Garlic, Minced

2 Teaspoon Rock Flavored Vinegar

2 Tablespoons Thyme, Fresh

2 Tablespoons Parsley, Fresh

2 Teaspoon Black Pepper

1 Tablespoon Olive Oil

½ Cup Beef Broth

Directions:

Set your pot to sauté and heat up the tablespoon of oil.

Once it's hot add the beef in batches to brown on all sides, and then place your beef to the side.

Slice your cooked bacon and add it to the strips. Add the strips bac into the pot with your onion, and then brown for three minutes.

Throw in the remaining ingredients, and seal the lid.

Cook on high pressure for thirty minutes, and then allow for a natural pressure release for ten minutes. Enjoy warm.

Nutrition:

Calories: 416, Protein: 18 Grams, Fats: 18 Grams, Carbs: 12 Grams

Lobster Bisque

Preparation Time: 10 minutes | Cooking Time: 10 minutes | Servings: 4

Ingredients:

1 Teaspoon Black Pepper

1 Teaspoon Dill, Dried

32 Ounces Chicken Broth, Low Sodium

1 Tablespoon Butter

2 Shallots, Minced

1 Clove Garlic, Minced

1 Cup Celery, Diced

1 Cup Carrots, Diced

29 Ounces Tomatoes, Diced

½ Teaspoon Paprika

4 Lobster Tails

1 Pint Heavy Whipping Cream

Directions:

Add in the garlic, shallots and butter in a microwave safe bowl. Microwave for three minutes before adding in the tomatoes, celery, carrot, garlic and shallots. Add it all into your instant pot.

Add in the broth and spices, and then use a knife to cut the lobster tails.

Lock the lid and cook on high pressure for four minutes. Use a natural pressure release for ten minutes followed by a quick release.

Use an immersion blender, and blend until smooth.

Nutrition:

Calories: 437, Protein: 38 Grams, Fat: 17 Grams, Carbs: 21 Grams

Pineapple Spicy Shrimp

Preparation Time: 3 minutes | Cooking Time: 12 minutes | Servings: 4

Ingredients:

¼ Cup Dry White Wine

2 Tablespoons Soy Sauce

2 Tablespoon Thai Sweet Chili Sauce

1 lb. Shrimp, Large

1 Tablespoon Ground Chili Paste

½ Cup Pineapple Juice, Unsweetened - 12 Ounces Quinoa

1 Red Bell Pepper, Large & Sliced

Directions: Drain your juice from the pineapple, and set it to the side. Measure ½ a cup of juice out. Mix together the bell pepper, pineapple juice, rice, wine, chili sauce, soy sauce, chopped scallions and chili paste in the bottom of your instant pot. Put the shrimp on top before locking the lid. Cook on high pressure for two minutes before using a natural pressure release for ten minutes. Follow with a quick release. Serve garnished with pineapple chunks and scallions.

Nutrition:

Calories: 299, Protein: 8 Grams, Fat: 5 Grams, Carbs: 54 Grams

Seafood & Chickpea Pot

Preparation Time: 5 minutes | Cooking Time: 20 minutes | Servings: 4

Ingredients:

2 Cod Fillets

2 Cups Vegetable Broth

2 Tablespoons Black Pepper

1 lb. Shrimp

1 Cup Scallions, Chopped - 1 Carrot, Chopped

1 Cup Chickpea, Soaked & Drained

1 Tomato, Chopped for Garnish

¼ Cup Cheese for Garnish

Directions:

Throw in all ingredients into your instant pot, and then seal the lid. Cook on high pressure for twelve minutes. Allow for a natural pressure release for ten minutes before following it with a quick release. Top with cheese and tomatoes before serving. Cheddar cheese is recommended.

Nutrition:

Calories: 268 Protein: 14.5 Grams Fat: 4.2 Grams Carbs: 45 Grams

Chicken & Mushroom Stew

Preparation Time: 20 minutes | Cooking Time: 20 minutes | Servings: 4

Ingredients:

4 Cloves Garlic, Diced

2 Bay Leaves

7 Ounces White Button Mushrooms

1 ¾ lb. Chicken Breasts, Diced

1 Teaspoon Flavored vinegar

1 Brown Onion, Halved & Sliced

2 Tablespoons Olive Oil

¼ Teaspoon Ground Nutmeg

½ Teaspoon Black Pepper

1 Teaspoon Dijon Mustard

½ Cup Chicken Stock

1/3 Cup Sour Cream

1 Teaspoon Arrowroot Powder

3 Tablespoons Parsley, Fresh & Chopped

Directions:

Press sauté and add the oil. Once the oil is hot add the vinegar and onion, cooking for four minutes.

Add in the mushroom, bay leaves, chicken, nutmeg, garlic, stock cube, pepper, water and mustard. Stir well.

Seal the lid and cook on high pressure for one minute.

Use a natural pressure release for ten minutes and then finish with a quick release.

Take out a few tablespoons of liquid and mix it with the arrowroot powder, pour it in and allow it to thicken for three minutes.

Add in the sour cream, and stir well. Serve warm and garnished with parsley.

Nutrition:

Calories: 249, Protein: 18 Grams, Fat: 17 Grams, Carbs: 5 Grams

Side Dish Recipes

Apple & Barley Side

Preparation Time: 15 minutes | Cooking Time: 15 minutes | Servings: 4

Ingredients:

1 Cup Barley

2 Cups Water

1 Cup Pesto, Salt Free

1 Green Apple, Chopped

¼ Cup Celery, Chopped

Black Pepper to Taste

Directions:

Put the water, salt, pepper and barely in your instant pot, and then seal the lid. Cook on high pressure for twenty minutes before using a quick release and draining it. Add your apple, pesto, pepper and celery to the barley, and then toss. Serve warm.

Nutrition:

Calories: 200 Protein: 7 Grams Fat: 5 Grams Carbs: 14 Grams

Spinach Dip

Preparation Time: 10 minutes | Cooking Time: 10 minutes | Servings: 4

Ingredients:

1 Bunch Spinach Leaves, Torn

1 Scallion, Sliced

2 Tablespoons Mint Leaves, Chopped

¾ Cup Coconut Cream

Black Pepper to Taste

Directions:

Mix the scallion, mint, cream, spinach and black pepper together. toss well, and seal the lid.

Cook on high pressure for ten minutes, and then use a quick release.

Use an immersion blender to blend before serving.

Nutrition:

Calories: 200, Protein: 8 Grams, Fat: 3 Grams Carbs: 16 Grams

Rice & Endives

Preparation Time: 10 minutes | Cooking Time: 25 minutes | Servings: 4

Ingredients:

1 Tablespoon Olive Oil - 2 Scallions, Chopped

1 Tablespoon Ginger, Grated

3 Cloves Garlic, Minced

1 Teaspoon Chili Sauce

Black Pepper to Taste

1 Cup White Rice - 2 Cups Vegetable Stock

3 Endives, Trimmed & Chopped

Directions:

Press sauté and add the oil. Once it's hot add in the ginger, scallions, chili sauce and garlic. Stir while cooking for five minutes. Add the rice and stock, and stir again. Cover, and cook on high pressure for seventeen minutes. Add the endives and pepper, and stir well. Seal the lid and cook on high pressure for five minutes before using a quick release and serve warm.

Nutrition:

Calories: 200 Protein: 8 Grams Fat: 5 Grams Carbs: 16 Grams

Lentils & Peas

Preparation Time: 10 minutes | Cooking Time: 12 minutes | Servings: 6

Ingredients:

½ Cup Red Lentils

1 Tomato, Chopped

½ Cup Yellow Split Peas

1 ½ Cups Water

3 Cloves, Minced

1 Yellow Onion, Chopped

1 Teaspoon Cumin Seeds

1 Teaspoon Ginger, Grated

½ Teaspoon Turmeric Powder

Directions:

Mix your lentils, peas, tomato, water, garlic, onion, cumin, ginger, and turmeric. Stir well, and then seal the lid. Cook on high pressure for twelve minutes, and then sue a quick release. Serve warm.

Nutrition:

Calories: 202 Protein: 5 Grams Fat: 4 Grams Carbs: 14 Grams

Leeks & Fennel

Preparation Time: 10 minutes | Cooking Time: 15 minutes | Servings: 2

Ingredients:

1 Fennel Bulb, Chopped

½ Cup Vegetable Stock, Low Sodium

1 Tablespoon Olive Oil

1 Leek, Chopped

Black Pepper to Taste

Directions:

Mix your fennel, leek, oi, stock and pepper. Seal the lid and cook on high pressure for fifteen minutes.

Use a quick release and serve warm.

Nutrition:

Calories: 162, Protein: 7 Grams, Fat: 5 Grams, Carbs: 7 Grams

Summer Squash Ribbons with Lemon and Ricotta

Preparation Time: 20 minutes | Cooking Time: 0 minutes | Servings: 4

Ingredients:

2 medium zucchini or yellow squash

½ cup ricotta cheese

2 tablespoons fresh mint, chopped, plus additional mint leaves for garnish

2 tablespoons fresh parsley, chopped

Zest of ½ lemon

2 teaspoons lemon juice

½ teaspoon kosher salt

¼ teaspoon freshly ground black pepper

1 tablespoon extra-virgin olive oil

Directions:

Using a vegetable peeler, make ribbons by peeling the summer squash lengthwise. The squash ribbons will resemble the wide pasta, pappardelle.

In a medium bowl, combine the ricotta cheese, mint, parsley, lemon zest, lemon juice, salt, and black pepper.

Place mounds of the squash ribbons evenly on 4 plates then dollop the ricotta mixture on top. Drizzle with the olive oil and garnish with the mint leaves.

Nutrition:

Calories: 90, Total Fat: 6g, Saturated Fat: 2g, Cholesterol: 10mg, Sodium: 180mg, Potassium: 315mg, Total Carbohydrates: 5g. Fiber: 1g, Sugars: 3g, Protein: 5g, Magnesium: 25mg, Calcium: 105mg

Sautéed Kale with Tomato and Garlic

Preparation Time: 5 minutes | Cooking Time: 10 minutes | Servings: 4

Ingredients:

1 tablespoon extra-virgin olive oil

4 garlic cloves, sliced

¼ teaspoon red pepper flakes

2 bunches kale, stemmed and chopped or torn into pieces

1 (14.5-ounce) can no-salt-added diced tomatoes

½ teaspoon kosher salt

Directions:

Heat the olive oil in a wok or large skillet over medium-high heat. Add the garlic and red pepper flakes, and sauté until fragrant, about 30 seconds. Add the kale and sauté, about 3 to 5 minutes, until the kale shrinks down a bit. Add the tomatoes and the salt, stir together, and cook for 3 to 5 minutes, or until the liquid reduces and the kale cooks down further and becomes tender.

Nutrition:

Calories: 110 Total Fat: 5g, Saturated Fat: 1g Cholesterol: 0mg Sodium: 222mg, Potassium: 535mg Total Carbohydrates: 15g Fiber: 6g, Sugars: 6g Protein: 6g Magnesium: 50mg Calcium: 182mg

Roasted Broccoli with Tahini Yogurt Sauce

Preparation Time: 15 minutes | Cooking Time: 30 minutes | Servings: 4

Ingredients:

1½ to 2 pounds broccoli, stalk trimmed and cut into slices, head cut into florets

1 lemon, sliced into ¼-inch-thick rounds

3 tablespoons extra-virgin olive oil

½ teaspoon kosher salt

¼ teaspoon freshly ground black pepper

½ cup plain Greek yogurt

2 tablespoons tahini

1 tablespoon lemon juice

¼ teaspoon kosher salt

1 teaspoon sesame seeds, for garnish (optional)

Directions:

Preheat the oven to 425°F. Line a baking sheet with parchment paper or foil.

In a large bowl, gently toss the broccoli, lemon slices, olive oil, salt, and black pepper to combine. Arrange the broccoli in a single layer on the prepared baking sheet. Roast 15 minutes, stir, and roast another 15 minutes, until golden brown.

To Make The Tahini Yogurt Sauce

In a medium bowl, combine the yogurt, tahini, lemon juice, and salt; mix well.

Spread the tahini yogurt sauce on a platter or large plate and top with the broccoli and lemon slices. Garnish with the sesame seeds (if desired).

Nutrition:

Calories: 245, Total Fat: 16g, Saturated Fat: 2g, Cholesterol: 2mg, Sodium: 305mg, Potassium: 835mg, Total Carbohydrates: 20g, Fiber: 7g, Sugars: 6g, Protein: 12g Magnesium: 65mg Calcium: 185mg

Green Beans with Pine Nuts and Garlic

Preparation Time: 10 minutes | Cooking Time: 20 minutes | Servings: 4-6

Ingredients:

1 pound green beans, trimmed

1 head garlic (10 to 12 cloves), smashed

2 tablespoons extra-virgin olive oil - ½ teaspoon kosher salt

¼ teaspoon red pepper flakes - 1 tablespoon white wine vinegar

¼ cup pine nuts, toasted

Directions: Preheat the oven to 425°F. Line a baking sheet with parchment paper or foil. In a large bowl, combine the green beans, garlic, olive oil, salt, and red pepper flakes and mix together. Arrange in a single layer on the baking sheet. Roast for 10 minutes, stir, and roast for another 10 minutes, or until golden brown. Mix the cooked green beans with the vinegar and top with the pine nuts.

Nutrition:

Calories: 165 Total Fat: 13g Saturated Fat: 1g Cholesterol: 0mg

Sodium: 150mg Potassium: 325mg Total Carbohydrates: 12g Fiber: 4g

Sugars: 4g Protein: 4g Magnesium: 52mg Calcium: 60mg

Roasted Harissa Carrots

Preparation Time: 10 minutes

Cooking Time: 15 minutes

Servings: 4

Ingredients:

1 pound carrots, peeled and sliced into 1-inch-thick rounds

2 tablespoons extra-virgin olive oil

2 tablespoons harissa

1 teaspoon honey

1 teaspoon ground cumin

½ teaspoon kosher salt

½ cup fresh parsley, chopped

Directions:

Preheat the oven to 450°F. Line a baking sheet with parchment paper or foil. In a large bowl, combine the carrots, olive oil, harissa, honey, cumin, and salt. Arrange in a single layer on the baking sheet. Roast for 15 minutes. Remove from the oven, add the parsley, and toss together.

Nutrition: Calories: 120 Total Fat: 8g Saturated Fat: 1gCholesterol: 0mg

Sodium: 255mg Potassium: 415mg Total Carbohydrates: 13g Fiber: 4g

Sugars: 7g Protein: 1g Magnesium: 18mg Calcium: 53mg

Cucumbers with Feta, Mint, and Sumac

Preparation Time: 15 minutes

Cooking Time: 0 minutes

Servings: 4

Ingredients:

1 tablespoon extra-virgin olive oil

1 tablespoon lemon juice

2 teaspoons ground sumac

½ teaspoon kosher salt

2 hothouse or English cucumbers, diced

¼ cup crumbled feta cheese

1 tablespoon fresh mint, chopped

1 tablespoon fresh parsley, chopped - ⅛ teaspoon red pepper flakes

Directions:In a large bowl, whisk together the olive oil, lemon juice, sumac, and salt. Add the cucumber and feta cheese and toss well. Transfer to a serving dish and sprinkle with the mint, parsley, and red pepper flakes.

Nutrition: Calories: 85 Total Fat: 6g Saturated Fat: 2g Cholesterol: 8mg

Sodium: 230mg Potassium: 295mg Total Carbohydrates: 8g Fiber: 1g

Sugars: 4g Protein: 3g Magnesium: 27mg Calcium: 80mg

Cherry Tomato Bruschetta

Preparation Time: 15 minutes

Cooking Time: 0 minutes

Servings: 4

Ingredients:

8 ounces assorted cherry tomatoes, halved

⅓ cup fresh herbs, chopped (such as basil, parsley, tarragon, dill)

1 tablespoon extra-virgin olive oil

¼ teaspoon kosher salt

⅛ teaspoon freshly ground black pepper

¼ cup ricotta cheese

4 slices whole-wheat bread, toasted

Directions:

Combine the tomatoes, herbs, olive oil, salt, and black pepper in a medium bowl and mix gently. Spread 1 tablespoon of ricotta cheese onto each slice of toast. Spoon one-quarter of the tomato mixture onto each bruschetta. If desired, garnish with more herbs.

Nutrition: Calories: 100 Total Fat: 6g Saturated Fat: 1g Cholesterol: 5mg

Sodium: 135mg Potassium: 210mg Total Carbohydrates: 10g

Fiber: 2g Sugars: 2g Protein: 4g Magnesium: 22mg Calcium: 60mg

Roasted Red Pepper Hummus

Preparation Time: 15 minutes

Cooking Time: 0 minutes

Servings: 2 cups

Ingredients:

1 (15-ounce) can low-sodium chickpeas, drained and rinsed

3 ounces jarred roasted red bell peppers, drained

3 tablespoons tahini

3 tablespoons lemon juice

1 garlic clove, peeled

¾ teaspoon kosher salt

¼ teaspoon freshly ground black pepper

3 tablespoons extra-virgin olive oil

¼ teaspoon cayenne pepper (optional)

Fresh herbs, chopped, for garnish (optional)

Directions:

In a food processor, add the chickpeas, red bell peppers, tahini, lemon juice, garlic, salt, and black pepper. Pulse 5 to 7 times. Add the olive oil and process until smooth. Add the cayenne pepper and garnish with chopped herbs, if desired.

Nutrition:

Calories: 130

Total Fat: 8g

Saturated Fat: 1g

Cholesterol: 0mg

Sodium: 150mg

Potassium: 125mg

Total Carbohydrates: 11g

Fiber: 2g

Sugars: 1g

Protein: 4g

Magnesium: 20mg

Calcium: 48mg

Baked Eggplant Baba Ganoush

Preparation Time: 10 minutes

Cooking Time: 1 hour

Servings: 4

Ingredients:

2 pounds (about 2 medium to large) eggplant

3 tablespoons tahini

Zest of 1 lemon

2 tablespoons lemon juice

¾ teaspoon kosher salt

½ teaspoon ground sumac, plus more for sprinkling (optional)

⅓ cup fresh parsley, chopped

1 tablespoon extra-virgin olive oil

Directions:

Preheat the oven to 350°F. Place the eggplants directly on the rack and bake for 60 minutes, or until the skin is wrinkly.

In a food processor add the tahini, lemon zest, lemon juice, salt, and sumac. Carefully cut open the baked eggplant and scoop the flesh into the food processor. Process until the ingredients are well blended.

Place in a serving dish and mix in the parsley. Drizzle with the olive oil and sprinkle with sumac, if desired.

Nutrition:

Calories: 50

Total Fat: 4g

Saturated Fat: 1g

Cholesterol: 0mg

Sodium: 110mg

Potassium: 42mg

Total Carbohydrates: 2g

Fiber: 1g

Sugars: 0g

Protein: 1g

Magnesium: 7mg

Calcium: 28mg

White Bean Romesco Dip

Preparation Time: 10 minutes

Cooking Time: 0 minutes

Servings: 4

Ingredients:

2 red bell peppers, or 1 (12-ounce) jar roasted sweet red peppers in water, drained

2 garlic cloves, peeled

½ cup roasted unsalted almonds

1 6-inch multigrain pita, torn into small pieces

1 teaspoon red pepper flakes

1 (14.5-ounce) can no-salt-added diced tomatoes

1 (14.5-ounce) can low-sodium cannellini beans, drained and rinsed

1 tablespoon fresh parsley, chopped

1 teaspoon sweet or smoked paprika

1 teaspoon kosher salt

¼ teaspoon black pepper

¼ cup extra-virgin olive oil

2 tablespoons red wine vinegar

2 teaspoons lemon juice (optional)

Directions:

If you are using raw peppers, roast them following the steps (see *Tip*), then roughly chop. If using jarred roasted peppers, proceed to step 2.

In a food processor, add the garlic and pulse until finely minced. Scrape down the sides of the bowl and add the almonds, pita, and red pepper flakes, and process until minced. Scrape down the sides of the bowl and add the bell peppers, tomatoes, beans, parsley, paprika, salt, and black pepper. Process until smooth.

With the food processor running, add the olive oil and vinegar, and process until smooth. Taste, and add the lemon juice to brighten, if desired.

Nutrition:

Calories: 180

Total Fat: 10g

Saturated Fat: 1g

Cholesterol: 0mg

Sodium: 285mg

Potassium: 270mg Total Carbohydrates: 20g Fiber: 4g

Sugars: 3g Protein: 6g Magnesium: 40mg Calcium: 65mg

Roasted Cherry Tomato Caprese

Preparation Time: 15 minutes

Cooking Time: 30 minutes

Servings: 4

Ingredients:

2 pints (about 20 ounces) cherry tomatoes

6 thyme sprigs

6 garlic cloves, smashed

2 tablespoons extra-virgin olive oil

½ teaspoon kosher salt

8 ounces fresh, unsalted mozzarella, cut into bite-size slices

¼ cup basil, chopped or cut into ribbons

Loaf of crusty whole-wheat bread for serving

Directions:

Preheat the oven to 350°F. Line a baking sheet with parchment paper or foil.

Put the tomatoes, thyme, garlic, olive oil, and salt into a large bowl and mix together. Place on the prepared baking sheet in a single layer. Roast for 30 minutes, or until the tomatoes are bursting and juicy.

Place the mozzarella on a platter or in a bowl. Pour all the tomato mixture, including the juices, over the mozzarella. Garnish with the basil.

Serve with crusty bread.

Nutrition:

Calories: 250

Total Fat: 17g

Saturated Fat: 7g

Cholesterol: 31mg

Sodium: 157mg

Potassium: 425mg

Total Carbohydrates: 9g

Fiber: 2g

Sugars: 4g

Protein: 17g

Magnesium: 35mg

Calcium: 445mg

Italian Crepe with Herbs and Onion

Preparation Time: 15 minutes

Cooking Time: 20 minutes per crepe

Servings: 6

Ingredients:

2 cups cold water

1 cup chickpea flour

½ teaspoon kosher salt

¼ teaspoon freshly ground black pepper

3½ tablespoons extra-virgin olive oil, divided

½ onion, julienned

½ cup fresh herbs, chopped (thyme, sage, and rosemary are all nice on their own or as a mix)

Directions:

In a large bowl, whisk together the water, flour, salt, and black pepper. Add 2 tablespoons of the olive oil and whisk. Let the batter sit at room temperature for at least 30 minutes.

Preheat the oven to 450°F. Place a 12-inch cast-iron pan or oven-safe skillet in the oven to warm as the oven comes to temperature.

Remove the hot pan from the oven carefully, add ½ tablespoon of the olive oil and one-third of the onion, stir, and place the pan back in the oven. Cook, stirring occasionally, until the onions are golden brown, 5 to 8 minutes.

Remove the pan from the oven and pour in one-third of the batter (about 1 cup), sprinkle with one-third of the herbs, and put it back in the oven. Bake for 10 minutes, or until firm and the edges are set.

Increase the oven setting to broil and cook 3 to 5 minutes, or until golden brown. Slide the crepe onto the cutting board and repeat twice more. Halve the crepes and cut into wedges. Serve warm or at room temperature.

Nutrition:

Calories: 135

Total Fat: 9g

Saturated Fat: 1g

Cholesterol: 0mg

Sodium: 105mg

Potassium: 165mg

Total Carbohydrates: 11g Fiber: 2g

Sugars: 2g Protein: 4g Magnesium: 30mg Calcium: 20mg

Pita Pizza with Olives, Feta, and Red Onion

Preparation Time: 15 minutes

Cooking Time: 10 minutes

Servings: 4

Ingredients:

4 (6-inch) whole-wheat pitas

1 tablespoon extra-virgin olive oil

½ cup hummus (store-bought or *Roasted Red Pepper Hummus*)

½ bell pepper, julienned

½ red onion, julienned

¼ cup olives, pitted and chopped

¼ cup crumbled feta cheese

¼ teaspoon red pepper flakes

¼ cup fresh herbs, chopped (mint, parsley, oregano, or a mix)

Directions:

Preheat the broiler to low. Line a baking sheet with parchment paper or foil.

Place the pitas on the prepared baking sheet and brush both sides with the olive oil. Broil 1 to 2 minutes per side until starting to turn golden brown.

Spread 2 tablespoons hummus on each pita. Top the pitas with bell pepper, onion, olives, feta cheese, and red pepper flakes. Broil again until the cheese softens and starts to get golden brown, 4 to 6 minutes, being careful not to burn the pitas.

Remove from broiler and top with the herbs.

Nutrition:

Calories: 185

Total Fat: 11g

Saturated Fat: 2g

Cholesterol: 8mg

Sodium: 285mg

Potassium: 13mg

Total Carbohydrates: 17g

Fiber: 3g

Sugars: 3g

Protein: 5g

Magnesium: 18mg

Calcium: 91mg

Roasted Za'atar Chickpeas

Preparation Time: 5 minutes

Cooking Time: 1 hour

Servings: 8

Ingredients:

3 tablespoons za'atar

2 tablespoons extra-virgin olive oil

½ teaspoon kosher salt

¼ teaspoon freshly ground black pepper

4 cups cooked chickpeas, or 2 (15-ounce) cans, drained and rinsed

Directions: Preheat the oven to 400°F. Line a baking sheet with foil or parchment paper. In a large bowl, combine the za'atar, olive oil, salt, and black pepper. Add the chickpeas and mix thoroughly. Spread the chickpeas in a single layer on the prepared baking sheet. Bake for 45 to 60 minutes, or until golden brown and crispy. Cool and store in an airtight container at room temperature for up to 1 week.

Nutrition: Calories: 150

Total Fat: 6g Saturated Fat: 1g Cholesterol: 0mg Sodium: 230mg

Potassium: 182mg Total Carbohydrates: 17g; Fiber 6g Sugars: 3g

Protein: 6g Magnesium: 32mg Calcium: 52mg

Roasted Rosemary Olives

Preparation Time: 5 minutes

Cooking Time: 25 minutes

Servings: 4

Ingredients:

1 cup mixed variety olives, pitted and rinsed

2 tablespoons lemon juice

1 tablespoon extra-virgin olive oil

6 garlic cloves, peeled

4 rosemary sprigs

Directions:

Preheat the oven to 400°F. Line the baking sheet with parchment paper or foil. Combine the olives, lemon juice, olive oil, and garlic in a medium bowl and mix together. Spread in a single layer on the prepared baking sheet. Sprinkle on the rosemary. Roast for 25 minutes, tossing halfway through. Remove the rosemary leaves from the stem and place in a serving bowl. Add the olives and mix before serving.

Nutrition: Calories: 100 Total Fat: 9g Saturated Fat: 1g Cholesterol: 0mg

Sodium: 260mg Potassium: 31mg Total Carbohydrates: 4g Fiber: 0g

Sugars: 0g Protein: 0g Magnesium: 3mg Calcium: 11mg

Crispy Cinnamon Apple Chips

Preparation Time: 15 minutes

Cooking Time: 1 hour and 15 minutes

Servings: 4

Ingredients:

3 apples, thinly sliced crosswise, seeded

1 tablespoon ground cinnamon

1 teaspoon granulated sugar

¼ teaspoon kosher salt

Directions:

Preheat the oven to 275°F. Coat a baking sheet with cooking spray. In a large bowl, whisk together the cinnamon, sugar, and salt. Add the apple slices and toss to evenly coat. Line up the apple slices on the baking sheet and roast for 45 minutes, then flip each chip and roast for another 45 minutes, until dried and crispy. Once cooled, store in an airtight container or plastic bag for up to 7 days.

Nutrition:

Total Calories: 80 Total Fat: 0g Saturated Fat: 0g

Cholesterol: 0mg Sodium: 147mg Potassium: 155mg

Total Carbohydrate: 21g Fiber: 4g Sugars: 15g Protein: 0g

Coconut Date Energy Bites

Preparation Time: 10 minutes

Cooking Time: 0 minutes

Servings: 4

Ingredients:

12 pitted Medjool dates

½ cup unsweetened shredded coconut

½ cup chopped walnuts or almonds

1½ tablespoons melted coconut oil

Directions:

Place all the ingredients in a food processor and pulse until the mixture becomes a paste. Form 2-inch bites, place in an airtight container, and store in the refrigerator for up to 2 weeks.

Nutrition:

Total Calories: 110

Total Fat: 6g

Saturated Fat: 3g

Cholesterol: 0mg Sodium: 1mg Potassium: 151mg

Total Carbohydrate: 16g Fiber: 2g Sugars: 13g Protein: 1g

Roasted Root Vegetable Chips with French Onion Yogurt Dip

Preparation Time: 20 minutes

Cooking Time: 20 minutes

Servings: 6

Ingredients:

FOR THE ROASTED ROOT VEGETABLE CHIPS:

1 sweet potato

1 Yukon Gold potato

1 beet

3 tablespoons canola oil

¼ teaspoon kosher salt

FOR THE FRENCH ONION YOGURT DIP:

1 tablespoon canola oil

1 yellow onion, peeled and thinly sliced

3 cloves garlic, peeled and minced

1 cup nonfat plain Greek yogurt

1 tablespoon mayonnaise

1 teaspoon Worcestershire sauce

½ teaspoon ground black pepper

½ teaspoon onion powder - ¼ teaspoon kosher or sea salt

¼ teaspoon dried mustard powder, ⅛ teaspoon ground cayenne pepper

TO MAKE THE ROASTED ROOT VEGETABLE CHIPS:

Directions:

Preheat the oven to 425°F. Coat a large baking sheet with cooking spray.

Thinly slice the sweet potato, Yukon Gold potato, and beet with a mandoline. Be careful! Coat them in the canola oil and sprinkle with the salt. Roast for about 16 minutes, flipping after 8 minutes, until crispy and lightly browned.

TO MAKE THE FRENCH ONION YOGURT DIP:

Heat the canola oil in a skillet over medium-low heat. Add the onion and sauté for 8 to 10 minutes, until caramelized and brown. Stir in the garlic and cook until fragrant, about 1 minute. Transfer the mixture to a bowl and add the Greek yogurt, mayonnaise, Worcestershire sauce, black pepper, onion powder, salt, dried mustard powder, and cayenne pepper. Mix until combined. The chips are best when served immediately. The sauce will keep in the refrigerator for 5 days.

Nutrition: Total Calories: 168 Total Fat: 11g

Saturated Fat: 1g Cholesterol: 2mg Sodium: 266mg Potassium: 342mg

Total Carbohydrate: 13g Fiber: 1g Sugars: 5gProtein: 5g

Stovetop Cheese Popcorn

Preparation Time: 10 minutes

Cooking Time: 0 minutes

Servings: 15

Ingredients:

¼ cup canola oil

½ cup white or yellow popcorn kernels

3 tablespoons nutritional yeast

½ teaspoon kosher salt

Directions:

Heat the canola oil over medium-high heat in a large stockpot. Add the popcorn kernels and place a lid on the pot. Let cook, shaking the pot periodically, until the popping stops. Remove from the heat, transfer to a large bowl, and top with the nutritional yeast and salt, shaking the bowl to coat the hot popcorn.

Nutrition:

Total Calories: 54 Total Fat: 4g

Saturated Fat: 0g Cholesterol: 0mg Sodium: 77mg Potassium: 0mg

Total Carbohydrate: 5g Fiber: 1g Sugars: 0g Protein: 1g

Sweet & Salty Nut Mix

Preparation Time: 10 minutes

Cooking Time: 45 minutes

Servings: 6

Ingredients:

1 tablespoon chili powder

½ tablespoon ground cinnamon

½ tablespoon granulated sugar

1 teaspoon ground ginger

½ teaspoon kosher or sea salt

¼ teaspoon ground cayenne pepper (optional)

2 large egg whites

½ cup unsalted peanuts

½ cup unsalted almonds

¼ cup unsalted cashews

Directions:

Preheat the oven to 300°F. Coat a baking sheet with cooking spray.

In a small bowl, whisk together the chili powder, cinnamon, sugar, ginger, salt, and cayenne pepper, if using.

In a larger bowl, whip the egg whites until slightly frothy. Then, stir in the peanuts, almonds, and cashews. After the peanuts, almonds, and cashews are coated, stir in the spice mixture until combined.

Transfer to the baking sheet and spread them out evenly. Bake for 40 to 45 minutes, until slightly browned.

Once cooled, store in an airtight container or plastic bag for up to 2 to 3 weeks.

Nutrition:

Total Calories: 204

Total Fat: g16

Saturated Fat: 2g

Cholesterol: 0mg

Sodium: 227mg

Potassium: 257mg

Total Carbohydrate: 11g

Fiber: 3g

Sugars: 3g

Protein: 8g

Dessert Recipes

Easy Cinnamon Baked Apples

Preparation Time: 5 minutes

Cooking Time: 45 minutes

Servings: 4

Ingredients:

4 apples, cored, peeled, and sliced thin

½ tablespoon ground cinnamon

¼ cup brown sugar

¼ teaspoon ground nutmeg

Optional: 2 teaspoons freshly squeezed lemon juice

Directions:

Preheat the oven to 375°F. Place apples in a mixing bowl and gently mix all the other ingredients together. Put apples in a nonstick pan. Cover and place in the oven. Bake for 45 minutes, stirring at least once every 15 minutes. Once they are soft, cook for another few minutes to thicken the cinnamon sauce. Serve.

Nutrition: Total Calories: 117 Total Fat: 1g Saturated Fat: 0g

Cholesterol: 0mg Sodium: 4mg Potassium: 206mg

Total Carbohydrate: 34g Fiber: 5g Sugars: 28g Protein: 0g

Chocolate Cake In a Mug

Preparation Time: 5 minutes

Cooking Time: 1 minutes

Servings: 1

Ingredients:

3 tablespoons white whole-wheat flour

2 tablespoons unsweetened cocoa powder

2 teaspoons sugar

⅛ teaspoon baking powder

1 egg white - ½ teaspoon olive oil

3 tablespoons nonfat or low-fat milk -½ teaspoon vanilla extract

Cooking spray

Directions: Place the flour, cocoa, sugar, and baking powder in a small bowl and whisk until combined. Then add in the egg white, olive oil, milk, and vanilla extract, and mix to combine. Spray a mug with cooking spray and pour batter into mug. Microwave on high for 60 seconds or until set. Serve.

Nutrition: Total Calories: 217 Total Fat: 4g

Saturated Fat: 1g Cholesterol: 1mg Sodium: 139mg Potassium: 244mg

Total Carbohydrate: 35g Fiber: 7g Sugars: 12g Protein: 11g

Peanut Butter Banana "Ice Cream"

Preparation Time: 10 minutes

Cooking Time: 0 minutes

Servings: 4

Ingredients:

4 bananas, very ripe, peeled and sliced into ½-inch rings

2 tablespoons peanut butter

Directions:

On a large baking sheet or plate, spread the banana slices in an even layer. Freeze for 1 to 2 hours.

In a food processor or blender, puree the frozen banana until it forms a smooth and creamy mixture, scraping down the bowl as needed. Add the peanut butter, pureeing until just combined. For a soft-serve ice cream consistency, serve immediately. For a harder consistency, place the ice cream in the freezer for a few hours before serving.

Nutrition:

Total Calories: 153

Total Fat: 4g

Saturated Fat: 1g Cholesterol: 0mg Sodium: 4mg Potassium: 422mg

Total Carbohydrate: 29g Fiber: 4g Sugars: 15g Protein: 3g

Banana-Cashew Cream Mousse

Preparation Time: 55 minutes

Cooking Time: 0 minutes

Servings: 2

Ingredients:

½ cup cashews, presoaked

1 tablespoon honey

1 teaspoon vanilla extract

1 large banana, sliced (reserve 4 slices for garnish)

1 cup plain nonfat Greek yogurt

Directions:

Place the cashews in a small bowl and cover with 1 cup of water. Soak at room temperature for 2 to 3 hours. Drain, rinse, and set aside. Place honey, vanilla extract, cashews, and bananas in a blender or food processor. Blend until smooth. Place mixture in a medium bowl. Fold in yogurt, mix well. Cover. Chill in refrigerator, covered, for at least 45 minutes. Portion mousse into 2 serving bowls. Garnish each with 2 banana slices.

Nutrition: Total Calories: 329 Total Fat: 14g

Saturated Fat: 3g Cholesterol: 8mg Sodium: 64mg Potassium: 507mg

Total Carbohydrate: 37g Fiber: 3g Sugars: 24g Protein: 17g

Peach and Blueberry Tart

Preparation Time: 10 minutes

Cooking Time: 30 minutes

Servings: 6-8

Ingredients:

1 sheet frozen puff pastry

1 cup fresh blueberries

4 peaches, pitted and sliced

3 tablespoons sugar

2 tablespoons cornstarch

1 tablespoon freshly squeezed lemon juice

Cooking spray

1 tablespoon nonfat or low-fat milk

Confectioners' sugar, for dusting

Directions:

Thaw puff pastry at room temperature for at least 30 minutes.

Preheat the oven to 400°F.

In a large bowl, toss the blueberries, peaches, sugar, cornstarch, and lemon juice.

Spray a round pie pan with cooking spray.

Unfold pastry and place on prepared pie pan.

Arrange the peach slices so they are slightly overlapping. Spread the blueberries on top of the peaches.

Drape pastry over the outside of the fruit and press pleats firmly together. Brush with milk.

Bake in the bottom third of the oven until crust is golden, about 30 minutes.

Cool on a rack.

Sprinkle pastry with confectioners' sugar. Serve.

Nutrition:

Total Calories: 119

Total Fat: 3g

Saturated Fat: 1g

Cholesterol: 0mg

Sodium: 21mg

Potassium: 155mg

Total Carbohydrate: 23g Fiber: 2g Sugars: 15gProtein: 1g

Sriracha Parsnip Fries

Preparation Time: 10 minutes

Cooking Time: 25 minutes

Servings: 4

Ingredients:

1 pound parsnips, peeled, cut into 3 × ½-inch strips

1 tablespoon olive oil

1 teaspoon dried rosemary

Sriracha to taste

Salt and pepper to taste

Directions:

Preheat oven to 450°F. Mix parsnips, rosemary, and oil in a medium size bowl. Season with salt, pepper, and sriracha to taste and toss to coat. Lay parsnips on a baking sheet making sure the strips don't overlap. (If they are touching they will become mushy instead of crispy.) Bake for 10 minutes. Turn and roast until parsnips are browned in spots, 10 to 15 minutes longer. If you want them to be extra crispy, turn the broiler on for the last 2 to 3 minutes. Remove from oven and enjoy.

Nutrition: Total Calories: 112 Total Fat: 4g Saturated Fat: 1g

Cholesterol: 0mg Sodium: 12mg Potassium: 419mg

Total Carbohydrate: 20g Fiber: 4g Sugars: 5g Protein: 2g

Tortilla Strawberry Chips

Preparation Time: 10 minutes

Cooking Time: 25 minutes

Servings: 6

Ingredients:

15 strawberry

¼ tsp. cayenne

2 tbsps. organic extra virgin olive oil

12 whole wheat grain tortillas

1 tbsp. chili powder

Directions:

Spread the tortillas for the lined baking sheet, add the oil, chili powder, strawberry and cayenne, toss, introduce inside oven and bake at 350 0F for 25 minutes.

Divide into bowls and serve as a side dish.

Enjoy!

Nutrition: Calories: 199 Fat: 3 g

Carbs: 12 g Protein: 5 g Sugars: 7 g Sodium: 9.8 mg

Almond Rice Pudding

Preparation Time: 10 minutes

Cooking Time: 30 minutes

Servings: 3-4

Ingredients:

¼ c. sugar

1 tsp. vanilla

3 c. milk

1 c. white rice

¼ c. toasted almonds

Cinnamon

¼ tsp. almond extract

Directions:

Get the milk and rice together in a pan and boil and simmer it by lowering the heat for half an hour with the top on till the rice softens up a bit.

Take it off the burner and put in sugar, almond, vanilla and cinnamon.

Garish roasted almonds at the top and eat it warm.

Nutrition: Calories: 80 Fat: 1.5 g

Carbs: 16 g Protein: 1 g Sugars: 7 g Sodium: 121.4 mg

Sweet Potatoes and Apples Mix

Preparation Time: 10 minutes

Cooking Time: 1 hour and 10 minutes

Servings: 1

Ingredients:

1 tbsp. low-fat butter

½ lb. cored and chopped apples

2 tbsps. water

2 lbs. sweet potatoes

Directions:

Arrange the potatoes around the lined baking sheet, bake inside oven at 400 0F for an hour, peel them and mash them in the meat processor.

Put apples in the very pot, add the river, bring using a boil over medium heat, reduce temperature, and cook for ten minutes.

Transfer to your bowl, add mashed potatoes, stir well and serve every day.

Enjoy!

Nutrition: Calories: 140

Fat: 1 g Carbs: 8 g Protein: 6 g Sugars: 2.6 g Sodium: 493.3 mg

Sautéed Bananas with Orange Sauce

Preparation Time: 5 minutes

Cooking Time: 5 minutes

Servings: 4

Ingredients:

¼ c. frozen pure orange juice concentrate

2 tbsps. margarine

¼ c. sliced almonds

1 tsp. orange zest

1 tsp. fresh grated ginger

4 firm, sliced ripe bananas

1 tsp. cinnamon

Directions: Melt the margarine over medium heat in a large skillet, until it bubbles but before it begins to brown.   Add the cinnamon, ginger, and orange zest. Cook, while stirring, for 1 minute before adding the orange juice concentrate. Cook, while stirring until an even sauce has formed.   Add the bananas and cook, stirring carefully for 1-2 minutes, or until warmed and evenly coated with the sauce.   Serve warm with sliced almonds.

Nutrition: Calories: 164.3

Fat: 9.0 gCarbs: 21.4 g Protein: 2.3 g Sugars: 26 g Sodium: 100 mg

Caramelized Blood Oranges with Ginger Cream

Preparation Time: 10 minutes

Cooking Time: 15 minutes

Servings: 4

Ingredients:

2 tbsps. low sugar orange marmalade

1 tbsp. divided fresh grated ginger

4 c. peeled and sliced blood oranges

2 tbsps. brown sugar

Candied orange peel

½ c. coconut cream

Directions:

Begin by preheating the broiler.

In a small saucepan combine the orange marmalade and two teaspoons of the fresh ginger. Heat over low heat and stir until the mixture becomes slightly liquefied.

Place a thin layer of the oranges into the bottom of four large baking ramekins and then brush with the marmalade mixture. Repeat this step until all of the oranges have been used. Pour any remaining gingered marmalade over the tops of the ramekins.

Sprinkle each ramekin with brown sugar and place under the broiler for approximately 5 minutes, or until caramelized.

Serve warm garnished with coconut cream and candied orange peel, if desired.

To make the coconut cream: Take one can of pure, unsweetened coconut milk and place it in your refrigerator for 24 hours. Take the can out of the refrigerator and scoop out the thick cream that has settled on top. Place this in a bowl, along with one teaspoon of ginger and beat until creamy.

Nutrition:

Calories: 220.2

Fat: 10.7 g

Carbs: 32.4 g

Protein: 2.4 g

Sugars: 19.5 g

Sodium: 143.7 mg

Grilled Minted Watermelon

Preparation Time: 10 minutes

Cooking Time: 10 minutes

Servings: 4

Ingredients:

1 tbsp. honey

¼ c. finely chopped fresh mint

8 thick deseeded watermelon slices

Directions:

Prepare and preheat a stovetop grill.

Lightly press towels against the watermelon slices to remove as much excess moisture as possible.

Lightly brush both sides of the watermelon slices with honey.

Place the watermelon slices on the grill and grill for approximately 3 minutes per side, or until slightly caramelized.

Serve warm, sprinkled with fresh mint.

Nutrition:

Calories: 199.2.

Fat: 2.6 g Carbs: 45.7 g Protein: 3.8 g Sugars: 10.4 g Sodium: 219.8 mg

Caramelized Apricot Pots

Preparation Time: 10 minutes

Cooking Time: 5 minutes

Servings: 6

Ingredients:

¼ c. white sugar

2 tsps. lemon juice

½ tsp. thyme

3 c. sliced apricots

1 tbsp. brown sugar

1 c. part skim ricotta cheese

1 tsp. lemon zest

Directions:

Preheat the broiler of your oven.

Place the apricots in a bowl and toss with the lemon juice.

In another bowl, combine the ricotta cheese, thyme, and lemon zest. Mix well.

Spread a layer of the ricotta mixture into the bottoms of 6 large baking ramekins.

Spoon the apricots over the top of the ricotta cheese in each.

Combine the white sugar and brown sugar. Sprinkle evenly over the apricots, avoiding large clumps of sugar as much as possible.

Place the ramekins under the broiler for approximately 5 minutes, or until caramelized.

Serve warm.

Nutrition:

Calories: 133.6

Fat: 3.6 g

Carbs: 21.6 g

Protein: 5.8 g

Sugars: 6 g

Sodium: 206 mg

Melon Mojito Granita

Preparation Time: 10 minutes

Cooking Time: 0 minutes

Servings: 6

Ingredients:

¼ c. chopped fresh mint

¼ c. lime juice

4 c. cubed cantaloupe melon

1 c. peach nectar

Directions:

Combine the melon, peach nectar, lime juice, and mint in a blender or food processor. Blend until smooth.

Place the mixture in a shallow metal pan and place in the freezer.

Check the mixture every 30 minutes or so. Using a spoon or fork, mix and scrape the mixture at every check, until a slushy ice has formed. This will take a couple of hours.

Take out of the freezer and let soften slightly before serving.

Serve with fresh fruit, if desired.

Nutrition:

Calories: 55.7 Fat: 0 g Carbs: 13.8 g Protein: 0.8 g Sugars: 12.5 g Sodium: 3 mg

Mocha Pops

Preparation Time: 10 minutes

Cooking Time: 0 minutes

Servings: 4-6

Ingredients:

½ tsp. pure vanilla extract

2 tbsps. honey

½ c. chopped almonds

¼ c. cooled brewed espresso

2 c. coconut milk

2 tbsps. dark cocoa powder

Directions:

In a blender, combine the coconut milk, honey, cocoa powder, espresso, and vanilla extract. Blend until creamy.

Pour the mixture into freeze pop molds and sprinkle with almonds.

Place in the freezer and freeze for at least 4 hours before enjoying.

Nutrition:

Calories: 317.3, Fat: 27.3 g Carbs: 17.3 g Protein: 4.6 g Sugars: 5 g Sodium: 26 mg

Rhubarb Pie

Preparation Time: 10 minutes

Cooking Time: 20 minutes

Servings: 12

Ingredients:

4 c. chopped rhubarb

8 oz. low-fat cream cheese

1 c. melted low-fat butter

1 ¼ c. coconut sugar

2 c. whole wheat flour

1 c. chopped pecans

1 c. sliced strawberries

Directions:

In a bowl, combine the flour while using the butter, pecans and ¼ cup sugar and stir well. Transfer this for some pie pan, press well in for the pan, introduce inside the oven and bake at 350 0F for 20 minutes. In a pan, combine the strawberries with all the current rhubarb, cream cheese and 1 cup sugar, stir well and cook over medium heat for 4 minutes. Spread this inside the pie crust whilst inside fridge for the couple hours before slicing and serving. Enjoy!

Nutrition:

Calories: 162, Fat: 5 g Carbs: 15 g Protein: 6 g Sugars: 16.6 g Sodium: 411 mg

Berry No Bake Bars

Preparation Time: 10 minutes

Cooking Time: 0 minutes

Servings: 18

Ingredients:

1 c. natural peanut butter

¼ c. chopped dried blueberries

3 c. oatmeal

¼ c. chopped dried cranberries

3 tbsps. honey

Directions:

Line a baking pan with wax paper or parchment paper.

Microwave the peanut butter for 10-15 seconds, just until it softens and begins to liquefy. Combine the oatmeal, peanut butter, honey, cranberries, and blueberries together in a bowl and mix until blended. Spread the mixture out evenly into the pan. Place in the refrigerator and let set for 2 hours before cutting into squares.

Nutrition:

Calories: 145.0 Fat: 6.4 g Carbs: 17.9 g Protein: 4.4 g Sugars: 17.9 g Sodium: 102.4 mg

Tropical Fruit Napoleon

Preparation Time: 20 minutes

Cooking Time: 0 minutes

Servings: 6-8

Ingredients:

1 tbsp. finely chopped fresh lemongrass

1 c. cubed mango

1 tsp. vanilla extract

1 peeled and cored whole pineapple

1 c. shredded unsweetened coconut

2 c. cubed papaya

2 c. light whipping cream

Directions:

Add the vanilla extract to the whipping cream and beat until thick and creamy. Fold in the coconut and lemongrass. Place in the refrigerator to chill for at least 30 minutes.

Cut the pineapple in thin, lengthwise pieces, creating "sheets" of pineapple.

Mix the mango and papaya together in a bowl.

Lay one-third of the pineapple sheets on a work surface

Spread a third of the whipping cream onto the pineapple.

Top with some mango and papaya. Follow this with another layer of pineapple, cream, and fruit.

Top with a final layer of pineapple, cream, and fruit.

Serve chilled and garnish with additional lemongrass, if desired.

Nutrition:

Calories: 128.5

Fat: 6.9 g

Carbs: 17.7 g

Protein: 1.0 g

Sugars: 6 g

Sodium: 80 mg

Ginger Peach Pie

Preparation Time: 10 minutes

Cooking Time: 45 minutes

Servings: 10

Ingredients:

5 c. diced peaches

½ c. sugar

2 refrigerated whole wheat pie crust doughs

1 tsp. cinnamon

½ c. orange juice

¼ c. chopped candied ginger

½ c. cornstarch

Directions:

Preheat the oven to 425°F.

Place one of the pie crusts in a standard size pie dish. Spread some coffee beans or dried beans in the bottom of the pie crust to use as a weight. Place the dish in the oven and bake for 10-15 minutes, or until lightly golden. Remove from the oven and let cool.

Combine the peaches, candied ginger, and cinnamon in a bowl. Toss to mix.

Combine the sugar, cornstarch, and orange juice in a saucepan and heat over medium until syrup begins to thicken.

Pour the syrup over the peaches and toss to coat.

Spread the peaches in the pie crust and top with the remaining crust. Crimp along the edges and cut several small slits in the top.

Place in the oven and bake for 25-30 minutes, or until golden brown.

Let set before slicing.

Nutrition:

Calories: 289.0

Fat: 13.1 g

Carbs: 41.6 g

Protein: 3.9 g

Sugars: 22 g

Sodium: 154 mg

Mocha Ricotta Cream

Preparation Time: 10 minutes

Cooking Time: 0 minutes

Servings: 4

Ingredients:

2 c. part skin ricotta cheese

1 tbsp. espresso powder

Almond cookie crumbs

½ c. powdered sugar

1 tbsp. dark cocoa powder

1 tsp. pure vanilla extract

Directions:

Combine the ricotta cheese, powdered sugar, espresso powder, cocoa powder, and vanilla extract in a bowl.

Using an electric mixer, blend until creamy.

Cover and refrigerate for at least 4 hours.

Serve in individual dishes, garnished with cookie crumbs, if desired.

Nutrition:

Calories: 230.6 Fat: 9.9 g Carbs: 22.0 g Protein: 14.3 g Sugars: 3.2 g Sodium: 166 mg

Fresh Parfait

Preparation Time: 10 minutes

Cooking Time: 0 minutes

Servings: 6

Ingredients:

4 peeled and chopped grapefruits

2 tsps. grated lime zest

4 c. non-fat yogurt

2 tbsps. lime juice

1 tbsp. chopped mint

3 tbsps. stevia

Directions:

In a bowl, combine the yogurt using the stevia, lime juice, lime zest and mint and stir.

Divide the grapefruits into small cups, add the yogurt mix in each and serve.

Enjoy!

Nutrition:

Calories: 200 Fat: 3 g Carbs: 15 g Protein: 10 g Sugars: 20 g Sodium: 13 mg

Toasted Almond Ambrosia

Preparation Time: 10 minutes

Cooking Time: 20 minutes

Servings: 2

Ingredients:

½ Cup Almonds, Slivered

½ Cup Coconut, Shredded & Unsweetened

3 Cups Pineapple, Cubed - 5 Oranges, Segment

1 Banana, Halved Lengthwise, Peeled & Sliced

2 Red Apples, Cored & Diced

2 Tablespoons Cream Sherry

Mint Leaves, Fresh to Garnish

Directions:

Start by heating your oven to 325, and then get out a baking sheet. Roast your almonds for ten minutes, making sure they're spread out evenly. Transfer them to a plate and then toast your coconut on the same baking sheet. Toast for ten minutes. Mix your banana, sherry, oranges, apples and pineapple in a bowl. Divide the mixture not serving bowls and top with coconut and almonds. Garnish with mint before serving.

Nutrition:

Calories: 177 Protein: 3.4 Grams Fat: 4.9 Grams Carbs: 36 Grams Sodium: 13 mg Cholesterol: 11 mg

Apple Dumplings

Preparation Time: 10 minutes

Cooking Time: 30 minutes

Servings: 4

Ingredients:

Dough:

1 Tablespoon Butter

1 Teaspoon Honey, Raw

1 Cup Whole Wheat Flour

2 Tablespoons Buckwheat Flour

2 Tablespoons Rolled Oats

2 Tablespoons Brandy or Apple Liquor

Filling:

2 Tablespoons Honey, Raw

1 Teaspoon Nutmeg

6 Tart Apples, Sliced Thin

1 Lemon, Zested

Directions:

Turn the oven to 350.

Get out a food processor and mix your butter, flours, honey and oats until it forms a crumbly mixture.

Add in your brandy or apple liquor, pulsing until it forms a dough.

Seal in a plastic and place it in the fridge for two hours.

Toss your apples in lemon zest, honey and nutmeg.

Roll your dough into a sheet that's a quarter inch thick. Cut out eight-inch circles, placing each circle into a muffin tray that's been greased.

Press the dough down and then stuff with the apple mixture. Fold the edges, and pinch them closed. Make sure that they're well sealed.

Bake for a half hour until golden brown, and serve drizzled in honey.

Nutrition:

Calories: 178

Protein: 5 Grams

Fat: 4 Grams

Carbs: 23 Grams

Sodium: 562 mg

Cholesterol: 61 mg

Apricot Biscotti

Preparation Time: 25 minutes

Cooking Time: 25 minutes

Servings: 4

Ingredients:

2 Tablespoons Honey, Dark

2 Tablespoons Olive Oil

½ Teaspoon Almond Extract

¼ Cup Almonds, Chopped Roughly

2/3 Cup Apricots, Dried

2 Tablespoons Milk, 1% & Low Fat

2 Eggs, Beaten Lightly

¾ Cup Whole Wheat Flour

¾ Cup All Purpose Flour

¼ Cup Brown Sugar, Packed Firm

1 Teaspoon Baking Powder

Directions:

Start by heating the oven to 350, and then mix your baking powder, brown sugar and flours in a bowl.

Whisk your canola oil, eggs, almond extract, honey and milk. Mix well until it forms a smooth dough. Fold in the apricots and almonds.

Put your dough on plastic wrap, and then roll it out to a twelve inch long and three inch wide rectangle. Place this dough on a baking sheet, and bake for twenty-five minutes. It should turn golden brown. Allow it to cool, and slice it to ½ inch thick slices, and then bake for another fifteen minutes. It should be crispy.

Nutrition:

Calories: 291

Protein: 2 Grams

Fat: 2 Grams

Carbs: 12 Grams

Sodium: 123 mg

Cholesterol: 21 mg

Apple & Berry Cobbler

Preparation Time: 10 minutes

Cooking Time: 30 minutes

Servings: 4

Ingredients:

Filling:

1 Cup Blueberries, Fresh

2 Cups Apples, Chopped

1 Cup Raspberries, Fresh

2 Tablespoons Brown Sugar

1 Teaspoon Lemon Zest

2 Teaspoon Lemon Juice, Fresh

½ Teaspoon Ground Cinnamon

1 ½ Tablespoons Corn Starch

Topping:

¾ Cup Whole Wheat Pastry Flour

1 ½ Tablespoons Brown Sugar

½ Teaspoon Vanilla Extract, Pure

¼ Cup Soy Milk

¼ Teaspoon Sea Salt, Fine

1 Egg White

Directions:

Turn your oven to 350, and get out six small ramekins. Grease them with cooking spray.

Mix your lemon juice, lemon zest, blueberries, sugar, cinnamon, raspberries and apples together in a bowl.

Stir in your cornstarch, mixing until it dissolves.

Beat your egg white in a different bowl, whisking it with sugar, vanilla, soy milk and pastry flour.

Divide your berry mixture between the ramekins and top with the vanilla topping.

Put your ramekins on a baking sheet, baking for thirty minutes. The top should be golden brown before serving.

Nutrition:

Calories: 131

Protein: 7.2 Grams

Fat: 1 Grams

Carbs: 13.8 Grams

Sodium: 14 mg Cholesterol: 2.1 mg

Conclusion

Now you know everything you need to in order to enjoy the benefits of the DASH diet. There's no reason to just deal with hypertension, but remember that even with his dietary change, you will still need any medication prescribed to your by your doctor as well as you'll need to exercise regularly to maintain your health and reap the full benefits. With regular exercise and healthy eating, a dietary approach to stopping hypertension is manageable. Don't let hypertension rule your life. Take back control by first taking back control of your diet.

www.ingramcontent.com/pod-product-compliance
Lightning Source LLC
Chambersburg PA
CBHW080759300326
41914CB00055B/961